# PRIMARY FRCS
# MCQ PRACTICE EXAMS

# PRIMARY FRCS
# MCQ PRACTICE EXAMS

**Edited by**
**Mary L. Forsling BSc. PhD.**
**Timothy J. Chambers MB. BS. BSc. PhD. MRCPath**

**PASTEST SERVICE**
P.O. Box 81
Hemel Hempstead
Hertfordshire England

©1985 PASTEST SERVICE
304 Galley Hill, Hemel Hempstead, Hertfordshire
Tel: (0442) 52113

All rights reserved. No part of this publication may be reproduced, stored in a retrieval system, or transmitted, in any form or by any means, electronic, mechanical, photocopying, recording or otherwise without the prior permission of the copyright owner.

First published 1985
Reprinted 1986

**British Library Cataloguing in Publication Data**

**Primary FRCS practice exams.**
1. Medicine – Problems, exercises, etc.
I. Forsling M.L. II. Chambers T.J.
610'.246171    R834.5.

**ISBN 0-906896-17-7.**

Text prepared using an IBM Microcomputer
Phototypeset by Sellars Phototype using an interface.
Printed by Martins of Berwick.

# CONTENTS

EXAMINATION TECHNIQUE                               vii

MULTIPLE CHOICE QUESTIONS                            1
  Instructions                              1
  Practice Exam 1                           3
  Practice Exam 2                          18
  Practice Exam 3                          33
  Practice Exam 4                          48
  Practice Exam 5                          63

ANSWERS AND TEACHING EXPLANATIONS
  Practice Exam 1                          78
  Practice Exam 2                          90
  Practice Exam 3                         102
  Practice Exam 4                         114
  Practice Exam 5                         126

RECOMMENDED READING AND REFERENCE LIST              138

MCQ REVISION INDEX                                  139

---

**IMPORTANT NOTICE**

The format of the FRCS examination changed in September 1990. There are now two sections: Applied Basic Sciences and Clinical Surgery-in-General. The multiple choice questions in this book are still relevant to the new Applied Basic Sciences MCQ paper but there are now 90 questions to answer instead of 60. Full details can be obtained from the Royal College of Surgeons.

# EXAMINATION TECHNIQUE

Multiple Choice Questions are the most reliable, reproducible and internally consistent method we have of testing re-call of factual knowledge. Yet there is evidence that they are able to test more than simple factual re-call; reasoning ability and an understanding of basic facts, principles and concepts can also be assessed. A good MCQ paper will discriminate accurately between candidates on the basis of their knowledge of the topics being tested. It must be emphasised that the most important function of an MCQ paper of the type used in the Primary FRCS, is to rank candidates accurately and fairly according to their performance in that paper. Accurate ranking is the key phrase; this means that all MCQ examinations of this type are, in a sense, competitive.

**Technique**
The safest way to pass Primary FRCS is to know the answers to all of the questions, but it is equally important to be able to transfer this knowledge accurately onto the answer sheet. All too often, candidates suffer through an inability to organise their time, through failure to read the instructions carefully or through failure to read and understand the questions. First of all you must allocate your time with care. There are 60 questions to complete in 2½ hours; this means 2½ minutes per question or 10 questions in 25 minutes. Make sure that you are getting through the exam at least at this pace, or, if possible, a little quicker, thus allowing time at the end for revision and a re-think on some of the items that you have deferred.

You must read the question (both stem and items) carefully. You should be quite clear that you know what you are being asked to do. Once you know this, you should indicate your responses by marking the paper boldly, correctly and clearly. Take great care not to mark the wrong boxes and think very carefully before making a mark on the answer sheet. Regard each item as being independent of every other item, each refers to a specific quantum of knowledge. The item (or the stem and the item taken together) make up a statement. You are required to indicate whether you regard this statement as 'True'. Look only at a single statement when answering, disregard all the other statements presented in the question. They have nothing to do with the item you are concentrating on.

**Marking your answer sheets**
The answer sheet will be read by an automatic document reader, which transfers the information it reads to a computer. It must therefore be filled out in accordance with the instructions. A sample of the answer

## Examination Technique

sheet, together with the instructions, can be obtained from the Royal College. Study these instructions carefully, well before the exams, the invigilators will also draw attention to them at the time of the examination. You must first fill in your name on the answer sheet, and then fill in your examination number. It is critical that this is filled in correctly. At present, page numbers must also be filled in, but in the future, it is possible that newly-designed sheets may remove the need for this step.

As you go through the questions, you can either mark your answers immediately on the answer sheet, or you can mark them in the question book first of all, transferring them to the answer sheets at the end. If you adopt the second approach, you must take great care not to run out of time, since you will not be allowed extra time to transfer marks to the answer sheet from the question book. The answer sheet must always be marked neatly and carefully according to the instructions given. Careless marking is probably one of the commonest causes of rejection of answer sheets by the document reader. For although the computer operator will do his best to interpret correctly the answer you intended, and will then correct the sheet accordingly, the procedure introduces a possible new source of error. You are, of course, at liberty to change your mind by erasing your original selection and selecting a new one. In this event, your erasure should be carefully, neatly, and completely carried out.

Try to leave time to go over your answers again before the end, in particular going back over any difficult questions that you wish to think about in more detail. At the same time, you can check that you have marked the answer sheet correctly. However, repeated review of your answers may in the end be counter-productive, since answers that you were originally confident were absolutely correct, often look rather less convincing at a second, third or fourth perusal. In this situation, first thoughts are usually best and too critical a revision might lead you into a state of confusion.

### To guess or not to guess

Do not mark at random. Candidates are frequently uncertain whether or not to guess the answer. However, a clear distinction must be made between a genuine guess (i.e. tails for True, heads for False) and a process of reasoning by which you attempt to work out an answer that is not immediately apparent by using first principles and drawing on your knowledge and experience. Genuine guesses should not be made. You might be lucky, but if you are totally ignorant of the answer, there is an equal chance that you will be wrong and thus lose marks. This is not a chance that is worth taking.

## Examination Technique

Although you should not guess, you should not give in too easily. What you are doing is to increase as much as possible, the odds that the answer you are going to give is the correct one, even though you are not 100% certain that this is the case. Take time to think, therefore, drawing on first principles and reasoning power, and delving into your memory stores. Do not, however, spend an inordinate amount of time on a single item that is puzzling you. Leave it, and, if you have time, return to it. If you are 'fairly certain' that you know the right answer or have been able to work it out, it is reasonable to mark the answer sheet accordingly. There is a difference between being 'fairly certain' (odds better than 50:50 that you are right) and totally ignorant (where any response would be a guess). The phrase 'MCQ technique' is often mentioned, and is usually used to refer specifically to this question of 'guessing' and 'Don't know'. Careful thought and reasoning ability, as well as honesty, are all involved in so-called 'technique', but the best way to increase the odds that you know the right answers to the questions, is to have a sound basic knowledge of medicine and its specialties.

**Trust the examiners**
Do try to trust the Examiners. Accept each question at its face value, and do not look for hidden meanings, catches and ambiguities. Multiple Choice Questions are not designed to trick or confuse you, they are designed to test your knowledge of medicine. Don't look for problems that aren't there, the obvious meaning of a statement is the correct one and the one that you should read.

Candidates often try to calculate their score as they go through the paper; their theory is that if they reach a certain score they should then be safe in leaving several answer boxes blank without needing to take the trouble to think out answers. This approach is not to be recommended. No candidate can be certain what score he will need to achieve to obtain a pass in the examination, and everyone will overestimate the score he thinks he has obtained by answering questions confidently. The best approach is to answer every question honestly and to make every possible effort to work out the answers to more difficult questions. In other words, your aim should always be to obtain the highest possible score on the MCQ paper.

*Examination Technique*

To repeat the four most important points of technique:

(1) Read the question carefully and be sure you understand it.
(2) Mark your responses clearly, correctly and accurately.
(3) Use reasoning to work out answers, but if you do not know the answer and cannot work it out, indicate 'Don't know'.
(4) The best way to obtain a good mark is to have as wide a knowledge as possible of the topics being tested in the examination.

John Anderson MB. BS. FRCP.
The Medical School
Newcastle-upon-Tyne.


## ACKNOWLEDGEMENTS

The editors would like to give special thanks to the many people who contributed questions and advice during the compilation of this book and in particular to Professor J. Joseph MD. DSc. FRCOG. for all his help.

# MULTIPLE CHOICE QUESTION PAPERS

### INSTRUCTIONS

In order to help Primary FRCS candidates revise for this difficult examination we have tried to follow as closely as possible the content and format of the official examination. Each question has an answer and teaching explanation which should provide a good basis for successful revision.

We suggest that you work on each set of 60 multiple choice questions as though it was a real Primary FRCS examination. In other words time yourself to spend no more than 2½ hours on each practice exam and do not obtain help from books, notes or persons while working on each test. Plan to take this practice exam at a time when you will be undisturbed for a minimum of 2½ hours. Choose a well lit location free from distractions, keep your desk clear of other books or papers, have a clock or watch clearly visible with a rubber and 2 well sharpened grade B pencils to hand.

As you work through each question in this book be sure and mark a tick or cross (True or False) against the A... B... C... D... E... answer space below each question. If you do not know the answer then leave the answer space blank. Thus when you have completed the paper you can mark your own answers with the help of the answers and explanations given at the end of the book. Do not be tempted to look at the questions before sitting down to take each test as this will not then represent a mock exam.

When you have finished an exam be sure to go back over your answers until the 2½ hours is over. When your time is up you can then mark your answers and study the teaching explanations carefully so as to learn from your mistakes. Give yourself +1 for every correct answer −1 for every incorrect answer and 0 for an unanswered question. Put a mark clearly on the book wherever you put a wrong answer and this will help you with your final revision as the official exam grows near.

Good luck with your revision.

# PRACTICE EXAM 1

*60 QUESTIONS: Time allowed 2½ hours*

Indicate your answers with a tick or cross in the spaces provided.

1  **The mandible**

    A  contains 10 erupted teeth at the age of 4 years
    B  is in direct contact with the lingual nerve
    C  is formed from the cartilage of the 2nd pharyngeal arch
    D  ossifies wholly in cartilage
    E  articulates directly with the temporal bone

    *Your answers:* A........ B........ C........ D........ E........

2  **The left coronary artery**

    A  gives off an anterior interventricular branch
    B  has no anastomoses with the right coronary artery
    C  gives off a circumflex branch which lies in the coronary (atrioventricular) sulcus
    D  gives off a posterior interventricular branch
    E  usually supplies the atrioventricular node

    *Your answers:* A........ B........ C........ D........ E........

3  **The brachial plexus gives off**

    A  the long thoracic nerve (nerve to the serratus anterior muscle) from its upper trunk
    B  the suprascapular nerve from its roots
    C  the musculocutaneous nerve from its medial cord
    D  the subscapular nerves from its posterior cord
    E  the radial nerve from its posterior cord

    *Your answers:* A........ B........ C........ D........ E........

4  **The arterial blood supply of the stomach**

    A  comes entirely from branches of the coeliac trunk
    B  includes the short gastric arteries which lie in the lienorenal ligament
    C  includes the right gastric artery, a direct branch of the coeliac artery
    D  along its greater curvature is by the left gastric artery
    E  includes branches of the hepatic artery

    *Your answers:* A........ B........ C........ D........ E........

*Practice Exam 1*

5  **The rectum**

   A  is a boundary of the ischiorectal fossa
   B  on its upper third is covered posteriorly by peritoneum
   C  has appendices epiploicae
   D  has taenia coli
   E  is a derivative of the hindgut

   *Your answers: A....... B....... C....... D....... E.......*

6  **The oesophagus**

   A  begins at the level of the 4th cervical vertebra
   B  is narrowed by the right bronchus
   C  is posterior to the left atrium
   D  passes through the diaphragm about 40 cm from the incisor teeth
   E  is posterior to the thoracic duct

   *Your answers: A....... B....... C....... D....... E.......*

7  **The sympathetic nervous system supplies**

   A  dilatator fibres to the coronary arteries
   B  constrictor fibres to the smooth muscle of the bronchial tree
   C  grey rami communicantes to the thoracic spinal nerves
   D  cholinergic secretomotor fibres to sweat glands
   E  fibres which cause the pupil to constrict

   *Your answers: A....... B....... C....... D....... E.......*

8  **The gall bladder**

   A  is related posteriorly to the superior (1st) part of the duodenum
   B  receives its arterial blood supply most commonly from the left hepatic artery
   C  is drained by a vein which ends in a hepatic vein
   D  has a fundus whose surface marking is where the lateral edge of the right rectus sheath meets the costal margin
   E  has a lining epithelium containing many goblet cells

   *Your answers: A....... B....... C....... D....... E.......*

*Practice Exam 1*

**9 The ulnar artery**

    A   passes superficial to the flexor retinaculum
    B   forms the major component of the superficial palmar arch
    C   lies lateral to the ulnar nerve
    D   passes deep to the flexor digitorum profundus muscle
    E   passes superficial to the pronator teres muscle

*Your answers: A....... B....... C....... D....... E.......*

**10 With regard to the bones of the wrist and hand**

    A   the metacarpals have already begun to ossify by the 12th week of fetal life
    B   the hamate has ossified by the 2nd year
    C   the capitate has not begun to ossify at birth
    D   the pisiform has ossified by the 8th year
    E   the scaphoid does not ossify until the 10th year

*Your answers: A....... B....... C....... D....... E.......*

**11 The hypoglossal nerve**

    A   is medial to the jugular foramen at the base of the skull
    B   is superficial to the hyoglossus muscle
    C   is superficial to the lingual artery
    D   supplies all the extrinsic muscles of the tongue
    E   emerges from the medulla oblongata between the pyramid and olive

*Your answers: A....... B....... C....... D....... E.......*

**12 The central tendon of the perineum (perineal body) receives fibres from the**

    A   ischiocavernosus muscle
    B   bulbospongiosus muscle
    C   both levator ani muscles
    D   sphincter uretrae (external urethral sphincter)
    E   external anal sphincter

*Your answers: A....... B....... C....... D....... E.......*

*Practice Exam 1*

**13 In the orbit the**

    A  ophthalmic artery is medial to the cone of muscles
    B  ophthalmic artery (or its branches) does not supply the retina
    C  ophthalmic veins have no valves
    D  ophthalmic veins drain into the cavernous sinus
    E  lacrimal gland is related to only the superior surface of the levator palpebrae superioris muscle

*Your answers: A....... B....... C....... D....... E.......*

**14 If the median nerve is cut just above the wrist**

    A  flexion at the interphalangeal joint of the thumb is lost
    B  the movement of opposition is lost
    C  there is loss of sensation in the nail bed of the index finger
    D  there is a loss of sensation in the skin over the thenar eminence
    E  there is a loss of abduction at the carpo-metacarpal joint of the thumb

*Your answers: A....... B....... C....... D....... E.......*

**15 In the autonomic nervous system the**

    A  pterygopalatine (sphenopalatine) ganglion is a relay station for neurons which supply the lacrimal gland
    B  grey rami communicantes contain preganglionic sympathetic fibres
    C  pelvic (inferior hypogastric) plexuses contain fibres which are from the thoracic and sacral autonomic outflows
    D  cardiac plexuses receive a contribution from all the cervical ganglia
    E  vagus nerve contains sympathetic preganglionic fibres

*Your answers: A....... B....... C....... D....... E.......*

**16 The inguinal canal in the female**

    A  has a floor formed by the inguinal ligament
    B  has the lacunar ligament in its floor laterally
    C  has the remains of the gubernaculum ovarii passing through it
    D  has the internal oblique in its roof
    E  has the conjoint tendon (falx inguinalis) in its posterior wall laterally

*Your answers: A....... B....... C....... D....... E.......*

## Practice Exam 1

**17 In the femoral triangle**

    A   the sartorius muscle lies laterally
    B   the adductor magnus muscle lies medially
    C   the pectineus muscle is in its floor
    D   the femoral nerve lies within the femoral sheath
    E   the great (long) saphenous vein passes through its roof

*Your answers: A....... B....... C....... D....... E.......*

**18 With regard to the meninges**

    A   the pia mater is very vascular
    B   the arachnoid mater in the adult extends to the level of the second sacral vertebra
    C   the pia mater forms the filum terminale
    D   the dura mater forms venous sinuses within the cranium
    E   the dura mater forms the ligamenta denticulata

*Your answers: A....... B....... C....... D....... E.......*

**19 In the 13 weeks old embryo**

    A   the pleuroperitoneal canals are still open
    B   the paramesonephric (Mullerian) ducts have partly fused
    C   the testes are in the inguinal canal
    D   the umbilical midgut loop has returned to the abdominal cavity
    E   haemopoiesis takes place mainly in the liver

*Your answers: A....... B....... C....... D....... E.......*

**20 In the posterior mediastinum**

    A   the upper three left posterior intercostal veins go to the left brachiocephalic vein
    B   the left lower posterior intercostal veins form the hemiazygos (inferior hemiazygos) vein
    C   the azygos vein joins the inferior vena cava
    D   the sympathetic trunk is posterior to the posterior intercostal veins
    E   the hemiazygos veins are posterior to the descending thoracic aorta

*Your answers: A....... B....... C....... D....... E.......*

*Practice Exam 1*

**21** In physiological terms the most logical form(s) of therapy of shock induced by severe burning of the skin is infusion of

    A   packed red blood cells
    B   whole blood
    C   plasma
    D   hypertonic sodium chloride
    E   hypotonic dextrose

*Your answers: A....... B....... C....... D....... E.......*

**22** The resistance to blood flow in a vessel

    A   depends on the thickness of the vessel wall
    B   is inversely proportional to the fourth power of the radius of the vessel
    C   is directly proportional to the length of the vessel
    D   is independent of haematocrit
    E   is directly proportional to the pressure drop along the vessel

*Your answers: A....... B....... C....... D....... E.......*

**23** The mean systemic filling pressure will be changed by

    A   increased total peripheral resistance
    B   contraction of skeletal muscles
    C   sympathetic stimulation
    D   haemorrhage
    E   posture

*Your answers: A....... B....... C....... D....... E.......*

**24** Pulmonary irritant receptors

    A   are located in the smooth muscle of the airways
    B   are found mainly in the bronchioles
    C   can be stimulated mechanically
    D   when stimulated initiate hyperpnoea and broncho-constriction
    E   have their information transmitted via myelinated vagal fibres

*Your answers: A....... B....... C....... D....... E.......*

*Practice Exam 1*

**25 Oxygen at high pressure may cause**

    A   brain damage
    B   nausea
    C   muscular twitching
    D   apnoea
    E   carbon monoxide to be driven off more quickly than normal

*Your answers: A....... B....... C....... D....... E.......*

**26 Lung compliance**

    A   is a measure of flow/pressure
    B   is measured under static conditions
    C   is dependent on lung size
    D   is increased in emphysema
    E   is increased in pulmonary fibrosis

*Your answers: A....... B....... C....... D....... E.......*

**27 The metabolic rate of the body can be increased as much as 40% by**

    A   shivering
    B   muscle activity
    C   catecholamines
    D   thyroid hormones
    E   insulin

*Your answers: A....... B....... C....... D....... E.......*

**28 Quantitatively which are the main buffers of hydrogen ions in the blood?**

    A   albumin
    B   haemoglobin
    C   phosphate
    D   bicarbonate
    E   ammonium ions

*Your answers: A....... B....... C....... D....... E.......*

*Practice Exam 1*

29 **Severe irritation of the mucosal lining of the small intestine leads to**

    A  a "peristaltic rush"
    B  failure of propulsion of chyme
    C  intestinal obstruction
    D  more rapid movement of chyme into the colon
    E  reduced motility to reduce the irritation

    *Your answers: A....... B....... C....... D....... E.......*

30 **The hunger contractions of the stomach**

    A  are associated with oesophageal and pyloric contractions co-existing in an empty relaxed stomach
    B  are increased by low blood sugar
    C  may occur in a totally vagotomised patient
    D  are only of a few seconds' duration
    E  occur only when the stomach has remained empty for a long period of time

    *Your answers: A....... B....... C....... D....... E.......*

31 **In patients with the Zollinger-Ellison syndrome**

    A  there is a pancreatic tumour
    B  a secretin releasing tumour is found
    C  characteristically there are recurrent peptic ulcers
    D  there is low basal gastric secretion
    E  there is additional release of gastrin by secretin

    *Your answers: A....... B....... C....... D....... E.......*

32 **The countercurrent multiplier system of the kidney**

    A  depends on the active transport of sodium
    B  involves the thick ascending limb of the loop of Henle being permeable to water
    C  is blocked by cooling the kidney to $0°C$
    D  produces a concentrated filtrate in the loop of Henle
    E  produces concentrated interstitial fluid in the medulla

    *Your answers: A....... B....... C....... D....... E.......*

## Practice Exam 1

**33** In secondary dehydration or hypotonic contraction there is experienced

    A   the sensation of thirst
    B   reduced urine volume
    C   a loss of salt in excess of water
    D   an increase in the intracellular fluid volume
    E   increased plasma protein concentration

*Your answers: A....... B....... C....... D....... E.......*

**34 Osmotic diuretics**

    A   produce a urine flow limited by the glomerular filtration rate
    B   retard absorption of salt and water
    C   include frusemide
    D   include sucrose
    E   include mannitol

*Your answers: A....... B....... C....... D....... E.......*

**35 Patients with excessive secretion of aldosterone may show**

    A   acidosis
    B   hypokalaemia
    C   hypertension
    D   weakness, usually episodic
    E   phosphaturia, polyuria and nocturia

*Your answers: A....... B....... C....... D....... E.......*

**36 In the control of diabetes mellitus**

    A   glycosuria is best controlled via very restricted dietary intake of carbohydrate
    B   exercise reduces the amount of insulin required
    C   weight reduction reduces the amount of insulin required
    D   the predisposition to arteriosclerosis is lessened if the control is via diet
    E   chlorpropamide may be of value

*Your answers: A....... B....... C....... D....... E.......*

## Practice Exam 1

**37 Thyroid binding globulin is increased by**

    A  pregnancy
    B  myxoedema
    C  acute porphyria
    D  nephrotic syndrome
    E  marked hypoproteinaemia

*Your answers: A....... B....... C....... D....... E.......*

**38 Prolactin secretion is inhibited by**

    A  PIF
    B  somatostatin
    C  TRH
    D  oxytocin
    E  increased plasma prolactin levels

*Your answers: A....... B....... C....... D....... E.......*

**39 A functioning cerebellum is important for**

    A  co-ordinating the movements involved in piano playing
    B  damping muscular movements
    C  initiating muscle movement
    D  maintaining smooth progression of movement
    E  predicting positions to be attained by moving limbs

*Your answers: A....... B....... C....... D....... E.......*

**40 Amongst receptors responding to mechanical deformation are**

    A  free nerve endings
    B  carotid baroreceptors
    C  Ruffini's endings
    D  Schwann cells
    E  Pacinian corpuscles

*Your answers: A....... B....... C....... D....... E.......*

## Practice Exam 1

**41 Haemolytic anaemia may be caused by**

    A  malaria
    B  high altitude
    C  abnormal haemoglobin
    D  iron deficiency
    E  glucose-6-phosphate dehydrogenase deficiency

*Your answers: A....... B....... C....... D....... E.......*

**42 Schaumann bodies may be seen in**

    A  chronic bronchitis
    B  mesothelioma
    C  sarcoidosis
    D  oat cell carcinoma
    E  tuberculosis

*Your answers: A....... B....... C....... D....... E.......*

**43 The following are primary neoplasms of bone**

    A  Wilms's tumour
    B  osteosarcoma
    C  osteophytoma
    D  trabecular carcinoma
    E  giant cell tumour

*Your answers: A....... B....... C....... D....... E.......*

**44 Plasma magnesium**

    A  if low, may cause tetany
    B  is reduced by steroids in primary hyperparathyroidism
    C  is often low in alcoholics
    D  falls in chronic renal failure
    E  may be reduced in malabsorption

*Your answers: A....... B....... C....... D....... E.......*

*Practice Exam 1*

## 45 Bacteroides

    A  are frequently killed by exposure to oxygen or desiccation
    B  are a minority component of the normal faecal flora
    C  are frequently involved in necrotic or gangrenous lesions
    D  are usually sensitive to metronidazole
    E  when found are frequently associated with other organisms

    *Your answers: A....... B....... C....... D....... E.......*

## 46 *Pseudomonas aeruginosa*

    A  is commonly present in human intestine
    B  is resistant to most antibiotics
    C  characteristically produces blue-green pus
    D  is typically transmitted in dust
    E  is a strict aerobe

    *Your answers: A....... B....... C....... D....... E.......*

## 47 Alpha-fetoprotein is commonly raised in

    A  adenocarcinoma of colon
    B  hepatoma
    C  neuroblastoma
    D  teratoma of testis
    E  hepatitis

    *Your answers: A....... B....... C....... D....... E.......*

## 48 Basophil adenoma of the pituitary

    A  may cause acromegaly
    B  may cause hypothyroidism
    C  may cause amenorrhoea
    D  occurs in the remnant of the craniopharyngeal duct
    E  may cause Cushing's syndrome

    *Your answers: A....... B....... C....... D....... E.......*

*Practice Exam 1*

**49** **The following antibodies are present in a previously untransfused group A rhesus negative patient**

    A    anti A
    B    anti B
    C    anti C
    D    anti D
    E    anti d

*Your answers: A....... B....... C....... D....... E.......*

**50** **Polycythaemia may be due to**

    A    adenocarcinoma of kidney
    B    hypersplenism
    C    Hodgkin's disease
    D    right-to-left shunts in the circulation
    E    Cushing's syndrome

*Your answers: A....... B....... C....... D....... E.......*

**51** **Primary gout is due to**

    A    increased tissue avidity for uric acid
    B    increased uric acid production
    C    debauchery and intemperance
    D    decreased uric acid destruction
    E    altered serum protein binding of uric acid

*Your answers: A....... B....... C....... D....... E.......*

**52** **The following are causes of cirrhosis**

    A    haemosiderosis
    B    galacatosaemia
    C    *S. mansonii*
    D    paroxysmal nocturnal haemoglobinuria
    E    chronic active hepatitis

*Your answers: A....... B....... C....... D....... E.......*

*Practice Exam 1*

**53 Syphilitic disease of the aorta is associated with**

   A  dissecting aneurysm
   B  perivascular plasma cells
   C  perivascular eosinophils
   D  aortic incompetence
   E  cystic medionecrosis

   *Your answers: A....... B....... C....... D....... E.......*

**54 The following statements are true of infectious mononucleosis**

   A  it can be caused by cytomegalovirus
   B  there is often a lymphocytosis
   C  anaemia is usual
   D  the heterophil antibody characteristic of the disease is absorbed by guinea-pig kidney
   E  the heterophil antibody is also absorbed by ox cells

   *Your answers: A....... B....... C....... D....... E.......*

**55 Intracerebral haemorrhage is associated with**

   A  Charcot-Bouchard microaneurysms
   B  benign essential hypertension
   C  rupture of middle meningeal artery
   D  multiple sclerosis
   E  hypokalaemia

   *Your answers: A....... B....... C....... D....... E.......*

**56 Left ventricular hypertrophy develops in**

   A  dextrocardia
   B  Fallots tetralogy
   C  coarctation of the aorta
   D  aortic stenosis
   E  mitral stenosis

   *Your answers: A....... B....... C....... D....... E.......*

*Practice Exam 1*

**57  In Duke's staging of colonic carcinoma**

    A  if the tumour is confined within the bowel wall at its site of origin it is stage A even if lymph nodes are involved
    B  the number of mitoses among tumour cell nuclei is assessed
    C  metastasis to distant organs is assessed
    D  stage A represents confinement of the tumour within the muscularis propria
    E  distance of tumour from resection lines is taken into account

    *Your answers:* A....... B....... C....... D....... E.......

**58  An increased incidence of atheroma is associated with**

    A  increased high density lipoprotein
    B  increased low density lipoprotein
    C  diabetes
    D  benign hypertension
    E  pulmonary hypertension

    *Your answers:* A....... B....... C....... D....... E.......

**59  *Actinomyces israelii***

    A  sometimes causes pelvic inflammatory disease
    B  is a gram positive aerobic organism
    C  is resistant to penicillin
    D  spreads via the lymphatics
    E  is a commensal in the caecum

    *Your answers:* A....... B....... C....... D....... E.......

**60  Polymorphonuclear leucocytes**

    A  proliferate in inflammatory sites
    B  are actively motile
    C  can produce IgD
    D  contain many lysosomal granules
    E  are actively phagocytic

    *Your answers:* A....... B....... C....... D....... E.......

END OF EXAM 1
Go over your answers until your time is up.
Answers and explanations are on page 78.

# PRACTICE EXAM 2

*60 QUESTIONS: Time allowed 2½ hours*
Indicate your answers with a tick or cross in the spaces provided.

1 **The radial artery**

   A   is medial to the radial nerve at the wrist
   B   is superficial to the tendon of extensor pollicis longus
   C   enters the palm by passing between the heads of the first dorsal interosseous muscle
   D   supplies arteries to all the digits
   E   is the main artery forming the deep palmar arch

   *Your answers: A....... B....... C....... D....... E.......*

2 **The following structures are derived from the midgut**

   A   the vermiform appendix
   B   the proximal third of the descending colon
   C   a persistent vitello-intestinal duct (or its remains)
   D   the distal third of the ascending colon
   E   the first part of the duodenum

   *Your answers: A....... B....... C....... D....... E.......*

3 **In the axilla**

   A   there are the trunks of the brachial plexus
   B   the axillary vein is medial to the artery
   C   the pectoralis major and minor muscles are in its lateral wall
   D   the serratus anterior muscle is in its medial wall
   E   the long thoracic nerve lies on its lateral wall

   *Your answers: A....... B....... C....... D....... E.......*

4 **The hypothalamus**

   A   forms part of the roof of the 3rd ventricle
   B   includes the tuber cinereum
   C   is part of the midbrain
   D   produces vasopressin
   E   is bounded anteriorly by the lamina terminalis

   *Your answers: A....... B....... C....... D....... E.......*

*Practice Exam 2*

## 5 The basilic vein

- A is a continuation of the ulnar side of the dorsal venous network of the hand
- B is deep to branches of the medial cutaneous nerve of the forearm at the elbow
- C is subcutaneous until it reaches the axilla
- D joins the cephalic vein to form the axillary vein
- E is separated from the brachial artery at the elbow by the bicipital aponeurosis

*Your answers: A....... B....... C....... D....... E.......*

## 6 In the orbit

- A the superior rectus muscle rotates the eyeball upwards and inwards
- B the superior oblique muscle rotates the eyeball inwards
- C the central artery of the retina enters the eyeball in the optic nerve
- D the levator palpebrae superioris muscle is supplied by both somatic and autonomic nerve fibres
- E the optic nerve is surrounded by an extension of two of the meninges

*Your answers: A....... B....... C....... D....... E.......*

## 7 The diaphragm

- A has a motor and sensory innervation
- B has a motor innervation from the 10th thoracic nerve
- C when paralysed moves upwards relative to the skeleton
- D is attached to the upper three lumbar vertebrae
- E is formed in part from the dorsal mesentery

*Your answers: A....... B....... C....... D....... E.......*

## 8 The serous pericardium

- A has a visceral layer which lines the fibrous pericardium
- B has an oblique sinus behind the right atrium
- C covers the ascending aorta and pulmonary trunk
- D has a transverse sinus posterior to the superior vena cava
- E forms the epicardium

*Your answers: A....... B....... C....... D....... E.......*

*Practice Exam 2*

9  **At the elbow**

   A  the radial nerve lies between the brachialis and brachioradialis muscles
   B  the joint is supplied by branches of the musculocutaneous, median and ulnar nerves and the nerve to the anconeus muscle
   C  the trochlear notch articulates with the capitulum
   D  the radial collateral (lateral) ligament is attached to the annular ligament
   E  the joint is supplied by branches from the ulnar, radial and profunda brachii arteries

   *Your answers: A....... B....... C....... D....... E.......*

10  **In the popliteal fossa**

   A  the biceps femoris muscle forms its upper lateral boundary
   B  the tibial (medial popliteal) nerve is deep to the popliteal artery
   C  the common peroneal (lateral popliteal) nerve is superficial to the lateral head of the gastrocnemius muscle
   D  the popliteus fascia forms part of the floor
   E  the popliteal vein is deep to the popliteal artery

   *Your answers: A....... B....... C....... D....... E.......*

11  **The deep perineal space (pouch) contains**

   A  branches of the pudendal nerve
   B  the bulbo-urethral (Cowper's) glands
   C  the bulbospongiosus muscle
   D  the corpora cavernosa
   E  the (external) sphincter of the urethra

   *Your answers: A....... B....... C....... D....... E.......*

12  **The ischiorectal fossa**

   A  contains the inferior rectal veins
   B  is bounded laterally by the ischium
   C  is bounded medially by the external anal sphincter
   D  has the pudendal (Alcock's) canal in its roof
   E  contains very little fat

   *Your answers: A....... B....... C....... D....... E.......*

*Practice Exam 2*

**13  If the common peroneal (lateral popliteal) nerve is divided**

    A   loss of sensation is limited to the big and little toes
    B   eversion of the foot is lost
    C   inversion of the foot is lost
    D   plantar flexion of the foot is lost
    E   dorsiflexion of the big toe is lost

*Your answers: A....... B....... C....... D....... E.......*

**14  The parotid gland**

    A   has a duct which opens into the floor of the mouth
    B   is innervated by the glossopharyngeal nerve
    C   is innervated by postganglionic fibres whose cell bodies are in the pterygo(spheno)palatine ganglion
    D   is related to the styloid process
    E   is related to the medial pterygoid muscle

*Your answers: A....... B....... C....... D....... E.......*

**15  The pelvic diaphragm**

    A   is partly fused with the longitudinal muscle of the rectum
    B   is attached to the obturator internus fascia
    C   has a bony attachment only to the pubic bone
    D   has fibres which enter the perineal body (central tendon of the perineum)
    E   contracts when coughing

*Your answers: A....... B....... C....... D....... E.......*

**16  The stomach**

    A   is anterior to the spleen
    B   is supplied posteriorly mainly by the left vagus nerve
    C   has secretomotor nerve fibres from sympathetic nerves
    D   has an oblique layer of muscle between its longitudinal and circular layers
    E   is separated from the splenic artery by the pancreas

*Your answers: A....... B....... C....... D....... E.......*

*Practice Exam 2*

17  **The ilio-inguinal nerve**

    A  is a branch of the 1st lumbar spinal nerve
    B  is sensory to the skin of the labia majora
    C  is a posterior relation of the kidney
    D  is entirely sensory
    E  passes through the deep inguinal ring

    *Your answers: A....... B....... C....... D....... E.......*

18  **The pelvic splanchnic nerves**

    A  come from the dorsal (posterior primary) rami of the 2nd, 3rd and 4th sacral spinal nerves
    B  are motor to the muscle of the sigmoid (pelvic) colon
    C  are necessary for erection of the penis
    D  are motor to the muscle of the vermiform appendix
    E  contain parasympathetic post-ganglionic fibres

    *Your answers: A....... B....... C....... D....... E.......*

19  **The aortic arch**

    A  is anterior and to the left of the bifurcation of the trachea
    B  passes upwards as far as the jugular (suprasternal) notch in the adult
    C  is crossed to its left (anteriorly) by the left phrenic nerve
    D  is joined in the fetus to the right pulmonary artery by the ductus arteriosus
    E  is anterior and to the left of the left recurrent laryngeal nerve

    *Your answers: A....... B....... C....... D....... E.......*

20  **The psoas major muscle**

    A  has the obturator nerve emerging from its medial border
    B  is crossed anteriorly by the gonadal vessels
    C  has the genitofemoral nerve emerging from its lateral border
    D  is medial to the external iliac vessels
    E  receives its nerve supply from the femoral nerve

    *Your answers: A....... B....... C....... D....... E.......*

*Practice Exam 2*

**21 Cardiac output**

    A   may be measured using the Fick principle and values for $O_2$ uptake, $PaO_2$ and $PvO_2$
    B   is about 1/10 of maximum when the subject is at rest
    C   does not alter with age
    D   is reflexly reduced on exposure to high temperature
    E   need not increase when heart rate increases

*Your answers: A....... B....... C....... D....... E.......*

**22 The child of a mother who had blood group A Rh positive and father AB Rh negative could be**

    A   A Rh positive
    B   B Rh positive
    C   AB Rh negative
    D   B Rh negative
    E   O Rh positive

*Your answers: A....... B....... C....... D....... E.......*

**23 A shift of oxygen - haemoglobin dissociation curve to the left is found with**

    A   anaemia
    B   cirrhosis of the liver
    C   hypothyroidism
    D   an increase of $H^+$
    E   an increase in $pCO_2$

*Your answers: A....... B....... C....... D....... E.......*

**24 Inhalation of 5% $CO_2$ at normal atmospheric pressure**

    A   increases hydrogen ion concentration in the cerebrospinal fluid
    B   through an effect on the oxygen dissociation curve reduces oxygen tension
    C   increases alveolar ventilation
    D   produces cutaneous vasoconstriction
    E   produces increased oxygen carriage by haemoglobin

*Your answers: A....... B....... C....... D....... E.......*

## Practice Exam 2

**25 The resistance of the airways**

 A is not constant in a given subject
 B comes largely from small peripheral airways
 C is increased by adrenaline
 D decreases in response to parasympathetic activity
 E is greater in inspiration than expiration

*Your answers: A....... B....... C....... D....... E.......*

**26 The work of inspiration**

 A represents about 4J (0.4kg.m) per minute
 B is effectively less as the result of surfactant
 C is increased in asthma because of narrowing of the bronchi
 D is greater if the elastic recoil of the lungs is greater
 E is less if inspiration starts at a higher than normal lung volume

*Your answers: A....... B....... C....... D....... E.......*

**27 Amongst the functions of plasma proteins are**

 A provision of metabolic fuel
 B control of plasma volume
 C a contribution to the immune response
 D transport of hormones
 E carriage of carbon dioxide

*Your answers: A....... B....... C....... D....... E.......*

**28 Adipose tissue cells**

 A contain triglycerides invariably with short chain fatty acids
 B contain less cholesterol than triglyceride
 C cannot convert glucose into triglyceride molecules, this transfer being restricted to the liver
 D contain glycerides in the liquid state
 E have a triglyceride content which turns over

*Your answers: A....... B....... C....... D....... E.......*

*Practice Exam 2*

**29 The cephalic phase of gastric secretion**

    A   begins when the food is tasted
    B   is mediated via the vagus
    C   involves some release of gastrin
    D   lasts no longer than 5 minutes
    E   does not alter mucous secretion

    *Your answers: A....... B....... C....... D....... E.......*

**30 Steatorrhoea can result from**

    A   coeliac disease
    B   partial gastrectomy
    C   deficient pancreatic secretion
    D   obstructive jaundice
    E   damage to liver cells

    *Your answers: A....... B....... C....... D....... E.......*

**31 Removal of large areas of the stomach can lead to**

    A   achlorhydria
    B   steatorrhoea
    C   megaloblastic anaemia
    D   a fall in plasma volume after a meal contributing to the dumping syndrome
    E   a rise in glucose concentrations contributing to the dumping syndrome

    *Your answers: A....... B....... C....... D....... E.......*

**32 Renal Blood flow**

    A   can be measured by a substance which is freely filtered
    B   can be measured using a substance which can be entirely removed from the glomerular filtrate
    C   is 1/5 to 1/4 of the total cardiac output
    D   falls in hard exercise
    E   varies directly with the blood pressure over the range 12-27 kPa (90-200 mm Hg)

    *Your answers: A....... B....... C....... D....... E.......*

*Practice Exam 2*

### 33 Excretion of drugs by the kidney

    A   may be an active process
    B   involves clearance rates of 0-600 ml/min
    C   is faster if the drugs are lipid soluble
    D   is faster if the drugs are non-ionic
    E   may be inhibited by compounds such as probenic acid

*Your answers: A....... B....... C....... D....... E.......*

### 34 If a very large volume of water is ingested

    A   the osmolality of the interstitial fluid will decrease
    B   the extra and intracellular fluid space will be expanded for at least 24 hours
    C   the activity of the neurohypophyseal neurones increases
    D   receptors in the carotid body will be stimulated
    E   right atrial receptors will be stimulated

*Your answers: A....... B....... C....... D....... E.......*

### 35 Adrenal corticosteroids

    A   include glucocorticoids
    B   include aldosterone
    C   are synthesized from cholesterol
    D   are secreted by the adrenal medulla
    E   are necessary for life

*Your answers: A....... B....... C....... D....... E.......*

### 36 Parathyroid hormone (PTH)

    A   is a glycoprotein
    B   is released in response to hypocalcaemia
    C   increases calcium reabsorption in the renal tubule
    D   increases phosphate reabsorption by the renal tubule
    E   acts directly on the intestine to promote calcium absorption

*Your answers: A....... B....... C....... D....... E.......*

*Practice Exam 2*

## 37  The hypothalamus

    A   synthesises hormones
    B   is the site of the pneumotaxic centre
    C   shows a common embryological origin with the posterior lobe of the pituitary
    D   is the site of thermal receptors
    E   influences anterior pituitary function via the portal blood system

*Your answers: A....... B....... C....... D....... E.......*

## 38  The criteria for a normal chemical transmitter include

    A   its storage in vesicles in the post-synaptic neurone
    B   the presence of enzymes for its synthesis in the synaptic cleft
    C   the absence from the synaptic area of enzymes capable of destroying the transmitter
    D   its release from presynaptic terminals when the action potential arrives at the terminal
    E   its being a peptide

*Your answers: A....... B....... C....... D....... E.......*

## 39  The knee jerk

    A   results from stimulation of the Golgi tendon organ
    B   is caused by stimulation of intrafusal fibres
    C   involves acetylcholine
    D   involves pre-synaptic excitatory potentials
    E   is unaffected by acute cerebellar lesions

*Your answers: A....... B....... C....... D....... E.......*

## 40  The retina in man

    A   possesses equal numbers of rods and cones
    B   has only rods in the central fovea
    C   has one blood supply via the central retinal artery
    D   receives an upright image of the field being viewed
    E   may be damaged by excessive illumination

*Your answers: A....... B....... C....... D....... E.......*

*Practice Exam 2*

**41 Leukaemia is associated with**

- A benzene poisoning
- B Down's syndrome
- C alcoholism
- D phenylbutazone therapy
- E deep X-ray therapy

*Your answers: A....... B....... C....... D....... E.......*

**42 Ureterocolic anastamosis may lead to**

- A metabolic alkalosis
- B hypochloraemia
- C hypokalaemia
- D hypernatraemia
- E increased renal bicarbonate excretion

*Your answers: A....... B....... C....... D....... E.......*

**43 The following drugs cause a dose-dependent suppression of bone marrow**

- A vincristine
- B benzene
- C mustine
- D phenylbutazone
- E penicillin

*Your answers: A....... B....... C....... D....... E.......*

**44 Which of the following are specific for Treponemal infection:**

- A W.R.
- B V.D.R.L.
- C Kahn
- D *Treponema pallidum* immobilisation test
- E fluorescent Treponemal antibody test

*Your answers: A....... B....... C....... D....... E.......*

*Practice Exam 2*

**45  Polycythaemia is associated with**

    A  clear cell carcinoma of the kidney
    B  methaemoglobinaemia
    C  cerebellar tumours
    D  gastric tumours
    E  breast tumours

*Your answers: A....... B....... C....... D....... E.......*

**46  Medullary carcinoma of thyroid**

    A  may produce thyroxine
    B  may be familial
    C  is hormone dependent
    D  is sometimes associated with phaeochromocytoma
    E  may show amyloid deposition

*Your answers: A....... B....... C....... D....... E.......*

**47  The following are caused by infection with *Streptococcus pyogenes***

    A  boils
    B  acute appendicitis
    C  rheumatic fever
    D  Sjogren's syndrome
    E  acute glomerulonephritis

*Your answers: A....... B....... C....... D....... E.......*

**48  Retinoblastoma**

    A  is sometimes hereditary
    B  is a form of teratoma
    C  is an optic melanoma
    D  is bilateral in a third of cases
    E  shows a similar histological appearance to medulloblastoma and neuroblastoma

*Your answers: A....... B....... C....... D....... E.......*

*Practice Exam 2*

**49 Thrombocythaemia is associated with**

    A   recovery from major surgery
    B   acute leukaemia
    C   a Schilling test in a patient with $B_{12}$ deficiency
    D   chronic granulocytic leukaemia
    E   polycythaemia rubra vera

*Your answers: A....... B....... C....... D....... E.......*

**50 Spirochaetes are associated with**

    A   Weil's disease
    B   Vincent's angina
    C   yaws
    D   syphilis
    E   trachoma

*Your answers: A....... B....... C....... D....... E.......*

**51 Berry aneurysms**

    A   are usually caused by atheroma
    B   are caused by syphilis in 20% of cases
    C   are due to congenital defects in the arterial media
    D   are only found in hypertensive patients
    E   are associated with polycystic renal disease

*Your answers: A....... B....... C....... D....... E.......*

**52 Carcinoma of the larynx**

    A   affects men considerably more often than women
    B   usually arises from the vocal cords themselves
    C   has a 5 year survival rate of about 10-30 per cent
    D   is an adenocarcinoma in 20% of cases
    E   shows a peak incidence in the fifth decade

*Your answers: A....... B....... C....... D....... E.......*

# Practice Exam 2

**53** The following are recognised associations of Down's syndrome

    A   trisomy of chromosome 21
    B   abnormal dermatoglyphic patterns
    C   atrial septal defects
    D   leukaemia
    E   webbing of the neck

*Your answers: A....... B....... C....... D....... E.......*

**54** The following organs typically demonstrate red infarction

    A   kidney
    B   lung
    C   small intestine
    D   myocardium
    E   spleen

*Your answers: A....... B....... C....... D....... E.......*

**55** Amyloid

    A   is a basophilic material stainable with Congo Red
    B   is often derived from a circulating protein precursor known as SAA
    C   may be a complication of histiocytosis X
    D   can be diagnosed by rectal biopsy
    E   shows a characteristic electron microscopical appearance

*Your answers: A....... B....... C....... D....... E.......*

**56** Teratomas

    A   occur most frequently in the gonads
    B   behaviour is related to HCG production
    C   rarely occur after the age of 15 years
    D   arise from totipotent cells
    E   are always malignant

*Your answers: A....... B....... C....... D....... E.......*

*Practice Exam 2*

**57 Hydrocephalus may be caused by**

A sagittal sinus thrombosis
B Arnold Chiari malformation
C cerebellar tumours
D parietal lobe infarction
E Gardner's syndrome

*Your answers: A....... B....... C....... D....... E.......*

**58 The agents of the following diseases have a non-human reservoir**

A yellow fever
B endemic typhus
C bubonic plague
D cholera
E leishmaniasis

*Your answers: A....... B....... C....... D....... E.......*

**59 Aspartate transaminase is raised in**

A myocardial infarction
B acute hepatitis
C acute pancreatitis
D Cushing's syndrome
E hyperthyroidism

*Your answers: A....... B....... C....... D....... E.......*

**60 Signs of ascites may be present in**

A Reye's syndrome
B Caplan's syndrome
C pseudomyxoma peritonei
D Pick's disease
E Meigs's syndrome

*Your answers: A....... B....... C....... D....... E.......*

END OF EXAM 2
Go over your answers until your time is up.
Answers and explanations are on page 90.

# PRACTICE EXAM 3

*60 QUESTIONS: Time allowed 2½ hours*

Indicate your answers with a tick or cross in the spaces provided.

1  Movements lost as a result of damage to the upper trunk of the brachial plexus (C5, 6) include

    A   abduction at the shoulder joint
    B   medial rotation at the shoulder joint
    C   extension at the shoulder joint
    D   pronation of the forearm
    E   flexion of the forearm at the elbow joint

*Your answers: A....... B....... C....... D....... E.......*

2  The glossopharyngeal nerve

    A   emerges from the skull through a foramen between the occipital and temporal bones
    B   contains motor fibres which supply the constrictor muscles of the pharynx
    C   contains preganglionic parasympathetic fibres which synapse in the submandibular ganglion
    D   is sensory to the carotid sinus
    E   contains taste fibres from the vallate (circumvallate) papillae

*Your answers: A....... B....... C....... D....... E.......*

3  The spermatic cord

    A   contains the genital branch of the genitofemoral nerve
    B   has a covering, the internal spermatic fascia, which is derived from the transversus abdominis muscle
    C   contains lymphatic vessels which go to the superficial inguinal lymph nodes
    D   contains lymphatic vessels which come from the scrotum
    E   is lateral to the pubic tubercle at the base of the superficial inguinal ring

*Your answers: A....... B....... C....... D....... E.......*

4  The tibial part of the sciatic nerve

    A   contains fibres supplying part of the biceps femoris muscle
    B   contains fibres supplying the abductor hallucis muscle
    C   gives branches to the knee joint
    D   gives off the saphenous nerve
    E   contains fibres supplying the lateral side of the foot

*Your answers: A....... B....... C....... D....... E.......*

*Practice Exam 3*

5  **The biceps femoris muscle**

  A  is deep to the common peroneal (lateral popliteal) nerve in the popliteal fossa
  B  is atached to the head of the fibula
  C  has an attachment to the linea aspera
  D  can laterally rotate the tibia at the knee joint
  E  is medial to the semimembranosus at their attachment to the ischial tuberosity

  *Your answers: A....... B....... C....... D....... E........*

6  **In the embryo at six weeks**

  A  the neural tube has closed
  B  herniation of part of the midgut is present
  C  the limb buds have already developed
  D  the palatine processes have fused
  E  the mandibular processes have fused

  *Your answers: A....... B....... C....... D....... E........*

7  **The deltoid muscle**

  A  is supplied by the 7th and 8th cervical spinal nerves
  B  is a flexor of the upper limb at the shoulder joint
  C  is the only muscle involved in the initiation of abduction of the upper limb at the shoulder joint
  D  is multipennate in the part attached to the clavicle
  E  can rotate the upper limb medially at the shoulder joint

  *Your answers: A....... B....... C....... D....... E........*

8  **The pituitary gland (hypophysis cerebri)**

  A  has an anterior lobe derived from the neural tube
  B  has a portal system of veins
  C  receives its arterial blood supply from the internal carotid artery
  D  is directly inferior to the optic nerves
  E  consists of cells derived from ectoderm

  *Your answers: A....... B....... C....... D....... E........*

## Practice Exam 3

**9  In the normal heart as it lies in the body**

A  the right border is formed by the right ventricle
B  the left border is formed by the left ventricle
C  the pulmonary artery is to the right of the ascending aorta
D  the left atrium is posterior
E  the apex is approximately 8 cm to the left of the midline in the 5th intercostal space

*Your answers: A....... B....... C....... D....... E.......*

**10  The radial nerve**

A  contains fibres from all the spinal nerves usually forming the brachial plexus (5th - 8th cervical and 1st thoracic)
B  supplies cutaneous branches to the back of the upper arm and forearm
C  gives a branch to the brachioradialis
D  contains fibres which innervate the skin of the back of the little finger
E  at the elbow lies in a groove between the brachialis and the biceps brachii muscles

*Your answers: A....... B....... C....... D....... E.......*

**11  With regard to the eyeball**

A  its nerve of general sensation is the ophthalmic division of the trigeminal nerve
B  its ciliary muscle is innervated by the oculomotor nerve
C  its postganglionic sympathetic fibres have their cell bodies in the inferior cervical ganglion
D  its postganglionic parasympathetic fibres have their cell bodies in the ciliary ganglion
E  its preganglionic sympathetic fibres have their cell bodies in the 1st thoracic segment of the spinal cord

*Your answers: A....... B....... C....... D....... E.......*

**12  In the ear**

A  the external acoustic (auditory) meatus can be staightened by pulling the pinna upwards and forwards
B  the skin of the external acoustic meatus receives a nerve supply from the vagus nerve
C  the tympanic membrane receives a nerve supply from the glossopharyngeal nerve
D  parts of the malleus and incus can be seen with the otoscope (auroscope)
E  the skin of the pinna receives a nerve supply from the mandibular nerve

*Your answers: A....... B....... C....... D....... E.......*

*Practice Exam 3*

## 13 The superficial perineal pouch contains

- A the (external) sphincter of the urethra
- B the crura of the clitoris
- C the greater vestibular glands (of Bartholin)
- D the bulbo-urethral glands (of Cowper)
- E the bulbospongiosus muscle

*Your answers: A....... B....... C....... D....... E.......*

## 14 The stomach

- A has branches of the splenic artery running along its greater curvature
- B is anterior to the omental bursa (lesser sac)
- C is posterior to the spleen
- D is supplied on its anterior surface mainly by the right vagus nerve
- E has branches of the hepatic artery running along its lesser curvature

*Your answers: A....... B....... C....... D....... E.......*

## 15 The prostate gland

- A has the opening of the utricle on the posterior wall of the prostatic urethra
- B has a stroma which is fibrous
- C has a median lobe lying between the urethra and the common ejaculatory ducts
- D has a uniform type of gland
- E has a venous plexus deep to its own capsule

*Your answers: A....... B....... C....... D....... E.......*

## 16 The dorsal (extensor) expansion of the middle finger

- A is attached to the middle and distal phalanges
- B has the 2nd lumbrical muscle attached to its lateral side
- C has the 2nd and 3rd dorsal interosseous muscles attached to it
- D has a synovial sheath
- E has the lumbrical muscle attached distal to the interosseous muscles

*Your answers: A....... B....... C....... D....... E.......*

*Practice Exam 3*

17  **The right coronary artery**

   A  arises from the anterior aortic sinus
   B  lies between the left atrium and pulmonary trunk
   C  supplies the sino-atrial node
   D  is distributed to only the right atrium and ventricle
   E  is smaller in calibre than the left coronary artery

   *Your answers: A....... B....... C....... D....... E.......*

18  **The midgut of the embryo and fetus**

   A  includes the whole of the duodenum
   B  is supplied by the superior mesenteric artery
   C  includes the transverse colon
   D  forms the umbilical hernia of the embryo and fetus
   E  undergoes a clockwise rotation

   *Your answers: A....... B....... C....... D....... E.......*

19  **With regard to approximate times of the eruption of some of the deciduous and permanent teeth**

   A  the deciduous lower central incisor erupts at about 6 months
   B  all the deciduous incisor teeth are present at the end of 1 year
   C  all the 8 permanent teeth in each quadrant are present by 16 years
   D  the deciduous incisor teeth are lost between 6 and 8 years
   E  the 2nd permanent molar is the 1st of the permanent teeth to erupt

   *Your answers: A....... B....... C....... D....... E.......*

20  **Preganglionic sympathetic nerve fibres**

   A  are found in peripheral nerves such as the median and ulnar nerves
   B  form the sympathetic plexuses surrounding blood vessels
   C  are present in the short ciliary nerves
   D  are found in the greater splanchnic nerves
   E  are non-myelinated

   *Your answers: A....... B....... C....... D....... E.......*

## Practice Exam 3

**21 The aortic valve**

    A  comprises two semilunar cusps
    B  has sinuses in the aortic wall superior to each cusp of the valve
    C  has chordae tendinae which prevents it prolapsing into the left ventricle
    D  when incompetent leads to a high pulse pressure
    E  when incompetent leads to low systolic pressure

*Your answers: A....... B....... C....... D....... E.......*

**22 A decrease in oxygen affinity of haemoglobin is found in**

    A  association with a fall in temperature
    B  association with an increase in red cell DPG
    C  residents at high altitude
    D  pregnancy
    E  association with an increase in pH

*Your answers: A....... B....... C....... D....... E.......*

**23 In the systemic capillaries**

    A  the blood flow rate is the same as in the aorta
    B  the concentration of chloride in red cells increases
    C  bicarbonate ions move out of red cells
    D  there is an increase in the affinity of haemoglobin for $O_2$
    E  the pH of blood falls

*Your answers: A....... B....... C....... D....... E.......*

**24 In the ECG of the adult**

    A  the QRS complex has the same duration as the ventricular systole
    B  the P wave coincides with depolarisation of the atria
    C  the R wave coincides with depolarisation of the apex of the heart
    D  the first heart sound occurs at about the same time as the P wave
    E  a P-R interval of 0.3 seconds indicates impaired conduction

*Your answers: A....... B....... C....... D....... E.......*

*Practice Exam 3*

## 25  Pulmonary surfactant

- A  is a lipoprotein material
- B  is produced in type 1 alveolar cells and excreted onto the surface of the alveoli
- C  does not appear until birth
- D  produces a constant surface tension
- E  if deficient or inactive leads to the neonatal respiratory distress syndrome

*Your answers: A....... B....... C....... D....... E.......*

## 26  The functional residual capacity

- A  is measured using a helium dilution method
- B  is approximately 1200 ml
- C  increases when lung recoil increases as in pulmonary fibrosis
- D  is reduced with increased airway resistance
- E  is the volume at which some airways normally begin to close during expiration

*Your answers: A....... B....... C....... D....... E.......*

## 27  The circulating volume of blood or plasma may be determined using

- A  $^{131}$I-labelled albumin
- B  labelled red cells
- C  rose bengal
- D  inulin
- E  deuterium oxide

*Your answers: A....... B....... C....... D....... E.......*

## 28  In very prolonged exercise

- A  blood glucose falls progressively
- B  plasma lactate concentrations fall progressively
- C  muscle glycogen stores are depleted
- D  gluconeogenesis is promoted by circulating catecholamines
- E  the tension of carbon dioxide in the arterial blood increases initially

*Your answers: A....... B....... C....... D....... E.......*

## Practice Exam 3

**29 Gluten-sensitive enteropathy**

    A  manifests itself as coeliac disease in children
    B  produces steatorrhoea in adults
    C  is associated with macrocytic anaemia
    D  is associated with impaired bile secretion
    E  cannot be treated as gluten is a very common food product

*Your answers: A....... B....... C....... D....... E.......*

**30 The effect of secretin on digestion is to**

    A  give a powerful stimulus to the secretion of pancreatic enzymes
    B  stimulate pancreatic bicarbonate secretion
    C  inhibit the action of gastrin
    D  stimulate bile secretion
    E  increase gastric motility

*Your answers: A....... B....... C....... D....... E.......*

**31 Segmentation in the small intestine**

    A  mixes chyme and moves it down the whole length of the intestine
    B  may be rhythmic and regularly spaced
    C  has a lower frequency in the upper part of the small intestine
    D  is under the influence of intramural nerves
    E  is inhibited by atropine

*Your answers: A....... B....... C....... D....... E.......*

**32 Glucose in the kidney**

    A  is filtered at the glomerulus and reabsorbed by the proximal tubule
    B  is secreted by the proximal tubule and reabsorbed by the distal
    C  is co-transported with sodium during reabsorption
    D  has its reabsorption potentiated by phlorizin
    E  can act as an osmotic diuretic

*Your answers: A....... B....... C....... D....... E.......*

*Practice Exam 3*

33  The extracellular fluid volume can be influenced by

    A    volume receptors in the cardiovascular system
    B    arterial pressure
    C    vasopressin
    D    aldosterone
    E    factor IV

*Your answers: A....... B....... C....... D....... E.......*

34  Under normal conditions the daily output in the urine includes approximately

    A    2.5 l water
    B    165 mmol $l^{-1}$ sodium chloride
    C    250 mmol $l^{-1}$ urea
    D    90 mmol $l^{-1}$ creatinine
    E    2.0 mmol $l^{-1}$ glucose

*Your answers: A....... B....... C....... D....... E.......*

35  The hormone insulin

    A    is produced in the pancreatic $\alpha$ cell
    B    increases the uptake of glucose by muscle
    C    facilitates protein synthesis
    D    facilitates glycogen synthesis
    E    stimulates release of non-esterified fatty acids from fat depots

*Your answers: A....... B....... C....... D....... E.......*

36  The action of steroid hormones in the target cells involves

    A    cell membrane receptors
    B    cytoplasmic receptors
    C    stimulation of adenylate cyclase
    D    increased active transport across the cell membrane
    E    increased synthesis of particular proteins

*Your answers: A....... B....... C....... D....... E.......*

*Practice Exam 3*

**37 Oral contraceptives (oestrogen and progesterone) act by**

    A  blocking the actions of endogenous oestrogen
    B  blocking the LH (luteinising hormone) surge
    C  preventing fertilisation of the ovum
    D  preventing embedding of the zygote
    E  producing abortion of the embedded fetus

*Your answers: A....... B....... C....... D....... E.......*

**38 In man vasopressin, the antidiuretic hormone**

    A  is synthesised in the supraoptic nucleus
    B  is released in response to reduced plasma volume
    C  acts to produce water retention
    D  is secreted at a constant rate throughout the 24 hours
    E  has a half time of 12 hours

*Your answers: A....... B....... C....... D....... E.......*

**39 In skeletal muscle**

    A  actin and tropomyosin are found in the thin filaments
    B  the thick filaments comprise myosin
    C  the lateral sacs of the sarcoplasm release Ca++
    D  troponin molecules bind Ca++
    E  the energy from ATP is used directly in force production

*Your answers: A....... B....... C....... D....... E.......*

**40 An uncomplicated transection of the spinal cord at the level of C5 in the long term results in loss of**

    A  a shivering reflex
    B  reflex micturition
    C  tendon jerks
    D  sweat gland activity below the level of the lesion
    E  abdominal reflexes

*Your answers: A....... B....... C....... D....... E.......*

*Practice Exam 3*

**41 The following statements are true of IgM**

    A  it is a polymer of IgG
    B  it is the commonest antibody in serum
    C  it is a major component of rheumatoid factor
    D  it can cross the placenta
    E  it is the earliest type of immunoglobulin to be produced following an antigenic stimulus

    *Your answers: A....... B....... C....... D....... E.......*

**42 Hypochromic microcytic red cells may be found in**

    A  thalassaemia minor
    B  pernicious anaemia
    C  iron deficiency
    D  chronic infection
    E  folate deficiency

    *Your answers: A....... B....... C....... D....... E.......*

**43 Hypercholesterolaemia may be caused by**

    A  biliary obstruction
    B  nephrotic syndrome
    C  hyperthyroidism
    D  hypothyroidism
    E  diabetes mellitus

    *Your answers: A....... B....... C....... D....... E.......*

**44** *Streptococcus pyogenes*

    A  is a synonym for $\beta$ haemolytic streptococci
    B  tends to arrange itself into clumps
    C  may produce erythrogenic toxin
    D  may cause erysipelas
    E  may be associated with erythema nodosum

    *Your answers: A....... B....... C....... D....... E.......*

*Practice Exam 3*

**45 The following statements are true of Herpes Zoster:**

    A  it is transmitted by direct contact
    B  it often occurs in small epidemics
    C  it is more common in patients with lymphoma
    D  it may be followed by chicken pox in contacts
    E  it is one cause of condylomata lata

    *Your answers: A....... B....... C....... D....... E.......*

**46 Adenolymphoma**

    A  is malignant lymphoma of salivary glands
    B  usually presents as a mass in the parotid region
    C  is commoner in men than women
    D  is also known as Warthin's tumour
    E  is a variant of pleomorphic adenoma

    *Your answers: A....... B....... C....... D....... E.......*

**47 The following are features of pyloric stenosis**

    A  low plasma bicarbonate
    B  low plasma chloride
    C  raised blood urea
    D  hyperkalaemia
    E  raised haematocrit

    *Your answers: A....... B....... C....... D....... E.......*

**48 Chronic lymphatic leukaemia is**

    A  associated with massive splenomegaly
    B  more common in females than males
    C  the commonest childhood leukaemia
    D  usually a neoplasm of B lymphocytes
    E  often associated with hypergammaglobulinaemia

    *Your answers: A....... B....... C....... D....... E.......*

*Practice Exam 3*

**49  Colonic diverticulosis**

    A   is caused by true diverticula
    B   is rare in the ascending and transverse colon
    C   is rare below the age of 40
    D   is associated with atrophy and fibrous replacement of the muscularis propria
    E   is considerably more common in females than males

*Your answers: A....... B....... C....... D....... E.......*

**50  T-Lymphocytes are the cell type responsible for**

    A   anaphylaxis
    B   serum sickness
    C   delayed hypersensitivity
    D   graft rejection
    E   Mantoux positivity

*Your answers: A....... B....... C....... D....... E.......*

**51  The following tumours are more common in children than adults**

    A   nephroblastoma
    B   glioblastoma
    C   medulloblastoma
    D   meningioma
    E   teratoma

*Your answers: A....... B....... C....... D....... E.......*

**52  Crohn's disease**

    A   may involve any part of the alimentary tract
    B   causes transmural inflammation
    C   frequently causes perforation
    D   only affects the colon if the ileum is also involved
    E   shows a recognised association with granulomas in many extra-alimentary organs

*Your answers: A....... B....... C....... D....... E.......*

*Practice Exam 3*

53 **The following is/are associated with a clinically significant increased risk of carcinoma**

    A    duodenal ulcer
    B    ileocaecal tuberculosis
    C    Crohn's disease
    D    polyposis coli
    E    diverticulosis coli

*Your answers: A....... B....... C....... D....... E.......*

54 **Adenocarcinoma of the prostate**

    A    spreads via the blood stream
    B    may regress after testosterone administration
    C    commonly produces osteosclerotic deposits in bone
    D    generally arises from anadenoma
    E    may cause gynaecomastia

*Your answers: A....... B....... C....... D....... E.......*

55 **The following is/are characteristically associated with the nephrotic syndrome**

    A    renal amyloidosis
    B    chronic pyelonephritis
    C    renal papillary necrosis
    D    Reye's syndrome
    E    cerebellar haemangioblastoma

*Your answers: A....... B....... C....... D....... E.......*

56 **The following are recognised causes of raised serum levels of creatine kinase**

    A    muscular exercise
    B    Duchenne's muscular dystrophy
    C    carriers of Duchenne's muscular dystrophy
    D    osteomalacia
    E    lead poisoning

*Your answers: A....... B....... C....... D....... E.......*

*Practice Exam 3*

## 57 Phenylketonuria

    A   causes a disease whose effects can be alleviated by reduction of dietary tyrosine
    B   causes severe mental retardation if untreated
    C   occurs approximately once in every thousand live births
    D   is a sex-linked recessive disease
    E   is an autosomal dominant disease

*Your answers: A....... B....... C....... D....... E.......*

## 58 Prolonged inhalation of silica dust characteristically causes

    A   pleural mesothelioma
    B   left ventricular hypertrophy
    C   carcinoma of bronchus
    D   retroperitoneal fibrosis
    E   fibrotic nodules in lung

*Your answers: A....... B....... C....... D....... E.......*

## 59 The following are true of tetanus

    A   the site of infection may be inconspicuous
    B   the causative organism has a characteristic 'drumstick' appearance
    C   infection spreads along fascial planes
    D   requires an anaerobic environment for germination of spores
    E   symptoms may commence months after infection

*Your answers: A....... B....... C....... D....... E.......*

## 60 Chronic lymphatic leukaemia

    A   often terminates in a 'blast crisis'
    B   is commonest in the third decade
    C   is frequently associated with deletion of part of chromosome 22
    D   sometimes causes swelling of lacrimal and salivary glands
    E   is more common in women than men

*Your answers: A....... B....... C....... D....... E.......*

END OF EXAM 3
Go over your answers until your time is up.
Answers and explanations are on page 102.

# PRACTICE EXAM 4

*60 QUESTIONS: Time allowed 2½ hours*

Indicate your answers with a tick or cross in the spaces provided.

1 **In swallowing**
 A the sensory side of the reflex is mediated by the glossopharyngeal nerve
 B the larynx is raised by the stylopharyngeus muscle
 C the nucleus ambiguus is involved
 D the vocal folds remain abducted
 E the aryepiglottis muscles contract

 *Your answers: A....... B....... C....... D....... E.......*

2 **With regard to the cerebellum**
 A the anterior (ventral) and posterior (dorsal) spinocerebellar tracts enter in the inferior peduncle
 B the fibres in the middle penduncle are mainly from the nuclei pontis
 C the fibres in the superior penduncles come mainly from the dentate nucleus
 D the oldest part of the cerebellum is associated with balance
 E the whole of the cortex has the same basic structure

 *Your answers: A....... B....... C....... D....... E.......*

3 **The rectus abdominis muscle**
 A has a sheath whose posterior wall is absent above the costal margin
 B is innervated by longitudinally running nerves
 C has tendinous intersections which are attached to the posterior layer of its sheath
 D forms the medial boundary of the inguinal (Hesselbach's) triangle
 E has on its posterior surface an arterial anastomosis connecting the subclavian with the external iliac arteries

 *Your answers: A....... B....... C....... D....... E.......*

4 **The lesser omentum**
 A contains a branch of the coeliac artery
 B contains the gastroduodenal artery
 C forms part of the anterior wall of the omental bursa (lesser sac)
 D contains the right and left gastric arteries
 E superiorly extends into the fissure for the ligamentum teres

 *Your answers: A....... B....... C....... D....... E.......*

## Practice Exam 4

**5 The obturator internus muscle**

- A has the pudendal nerve on its medial surface
- B has the obturator nerve on its medial surface
- C leaves the pelvis through the greater sciatic foramen
- D is a medial rotator of the thigh at the hip
- E is innervated by the 5th lumbar spinal nerve

*Your answers: A....... B....... C....... D....... E.......*

**6 In the eyeball**

- A the macula is medial to the optic disc
- B the aqueous humour is secreted by the ciliary processes
- C when the ciliary muscle contracts the suspensory ligament of the lens is relaxed
- D the pigment layer of the retina is firmly adherent to the rest of the retina
- E there are more rods than cones in the macula

*Your answers: A....... B....... C....... D....... E.......*

**7 The left phrenic nerve**

- A gives branches to the right crus of the diaphragm
- B is anterior to the left superior intercostal vein
- C is anterior to the terminal part of the thoracic duct
- D is posterior to the hilum of the lung
- E is superficial to the suprascapular artery on the scalenus anterior muscle

*Your answers: A....... B....... C....... D....... E.......*

**8 The inferior epigastric artery**

- A gives off a branch which goes to the spermatic cord
- B is medial to the deep inguinal ring
- C is medial to the obliterated umbilical artery
- D lies between the rectus muscle and the anterior layer of the rectus sheath
- E gives off an abnormal obturator artery when that is present

*Your answers: A....... B....... C....... D....... E.......*

*Practice Exam 4*

## 9 The first rib

- A has the scalenus medius muscle attached to the scalene tubercle
- B has the suprapleural membrane (Sibson's fascia) attached to its lateral border
- C has the stellate (cervicothoracic) ganglion anterior to its head
- D has the upper trunk of the brachial plexus directly related to its upper surface
- E has the superior intercostal artery anterior to its neck

*Your answers: A....... B....... C....... D....... E.......*

## 10 The female breast

- A has about 30-40 lobes
- B has a separate duct for each lobe
- C has suspensory ligaments (of Cooper) extending from the skin to the fascia covering the pectoralis major
- D has a nipple which contains a large number of sebaceous glands
- E develops a considerable amount of glandular tissue at puberty

*Your answers: A....... B....... C....... D....... E.......*

## 11 The vagina

- A has a posterior fornix closely related to the recto-uterine pouch of peritoneum
- B has lateral fornices closely related to the ureters
- C undergoes changes during the menstrual cycle
- D has an anterior wall related to a pouch of peritoneum
- E is partly developed from the urogenital sinus

*Your answers: A....... B....... C....... D....... E.......*

## 12 The median nerve

- A is lateral to the brachial artery at the elbow
- B is lateral to the axillary artery
- C is medial to the flexor carpi radialis muscle at the wrist
- D is deep to the flexor digitorum superficialis muscle in the forearm
- E has branches which are superficial to the superficial palmar arch in the palm

*Your answers: A....... B....... C....... D....... E.......*

## Practice Exam 4

**13  The obturator nerve**

    A  is lateral to the ureter in the pelvis
    B  is medial to the internal iliac artery
    C  leaves the pelvis through an opening in the lower part of the obturator membrane
    D  supplies the obturator internus muscle
    E  has an anterior branch which supplies only muscles

*Your answers:* A....... B....... C....... D....... E.......

**14  Structures passing through the foramen magnum include**

    A  the hypoglossal nerves
    B  the internal vertebral venous plexus
    C  the cranial accessory nerves
    D  the vertebral arteries
    E  the endosteal (outer) layer of the cranial dura mater

*Your answers:* A....... B....... C....... D....... E.......

**15  The sciatic nerve**

    A  is deep to the upper lateral part of the gluteus maximus muscle
    B  gives branches to the hamstring muscles
    C  is posterior to the quadratus femoris muscle
    D  gives an articular branch to the hip joint
    E  is medial to the posterior femoral cutaneous nerve

*Your answers:* A....... B....... C....... D....... E.......

**16  In movements of the scapula on the chest wall**

    A  the serratus anterior muscle pulls the scapula forwards
    B  the trapezius muscle pulls the scapula medially and backwards
    C  the rhomboid muscles rotate the scapula so that the glenoid cavity faces upwards (lateral rotation)
    D  the pectoralis minor muscle pulls the scapula forwards
    E  the pectoralis minor muscle rotates the scapula so that the glenoid fossa faces upwards (lateral rotation)

*Your answers:* A....... B....... C....... D....... E.......

*Practice Exam 4*

**17 In the femoral triangle**

    A  the pectineus muscle is lateral to the psoas tendon
    B  the femoral vein lies between the femoral artery and the femoral canal
    C  the femoral branch of the genitofemoral nerve lies within the femoral sheath
    D  the superficial epigastric vein joins the femoral vein
    E  the superficial epigastric artery passes through the saphenous opening

*Your answers: A....... B....... C....... D....... E.......*

**18 The right ureter**

    A  in the abdomen is anterior to the gonadal vessels
    B  in the abdomen is anterior to the ileocolic artery
    C  in the abdomen is posterior to the genitofemoral nerve
    D  in the pelvis is crossed internally (medially) by the obturator nerve
    E  enters the pelvis 3 cm lateral to the sacro-iliac joint

*Your answers: A....... B....... C....... D....... E.......*

**19 The femoral nerve**

    A  ends as a cutaneous nerve which runs along the lateral border of the foot
    B  is outside the femoral sheath
    C  gives off the lateral femoral cutaneous nerve
    D  supplies the pectineus muscle
    E  gives a sensory branch to the knee joint

*Your answers: A....... B....... C....... D....... E.......*

**20 In the development of the aortic arch arteries**

    A  a part of the sixth forms the ductus arteriosus
    B  a part of the fourth forms the subclavian artery
    C  a part of the third contributes to the internal carotid artery
    D  a part of the left sixth contributes to the pulmonary trunk
    E  the right sixth disappears completely

*Your answers: A....... B....... C....... D....... E.......*

## Practice Exam 4

**21** The systemic blood pressure

  A  increases invariably with increased heart rate
  B  decreases with age
  C  increases with sudden exposure to cold
  D  falls on assumption of the upright posture
  E  is increased by brain stem asphyxia

  *Your answers:* A....... B....... C....... D....... E.......

**22** Peripheral oedema may occur

  A  during pregnancy
  B  in very hot weather
  C  with arteriolar constriction
  D  with hepatic disease
  E  with reduced lymphatic drainage

  *Your answers:* A....... B....... C....... D....... E.......

**23** Intravascular clotting

  A  is induced with a decrease in blood flow
  B  does not occur as calcium is present
  C  occurs with accumulation of lipids and small muscle cells in arterial walls
  D  may be caused after childbirth by a rise in plasma fibrinogen
  E  is related to the clumping of platelets

  *Your answers:* A....... B....... C....... D....... E.......

**24** Vasodilatation is produced by

  A  vasopressin
  B  5-hydroxytryptamine (5HT)
  C  histamine
  D  bradykinin
  E  angiotensin

  *Your answers:* A....... B....... C....... D....... E.......

Practice Exam 4

**25** Voluntary hyperventilation can give rise to

  A  an alveolar $pCO_2$ of less than 5.3 kPa (40 mm Hg)
  B  an arterial pH of 7.3
  C  carpo-pedal spasm
  D  an increased renal excretion of acid
  E  increased cerebral blood flow

  Your answers: A....... B....... C....... D....... E.......

**26** Periodic or Cheyne-Stokes respiration may accompany

  A  hyperventilation
  B  pulmonary oedema
  C  ascent to high altitude
  D  decreased arterial $pO_2$
  E  increased circulation time

  Your answers: A....... B....... C....... D....... E.......

**27** The cells of the liver

  A  receive the greater part of their blood supply from the hepatic artery
  B  are the major site of urea formation
  C  are the major site of synthesis of immunoglobulins
  D  store vitamins A and D
  E  form glycogen from lactate

  Your answers: A....... B....... C....... D....... E.......

**28** Secretions of the exocrine pancreas

  A  come from the islets of Langerhans
  B  are rich in enzymes on stimulation by acetylcholine
  C  are copious in response to secretin
  D  can increase in response to a high pH in the duodenum
  E  are stimulated by protein digestion products

  Your answers: A....... B....... C....... D....... E.......

*Practice Exam 4*

**29  The ileum is the main site of absorption of**

    A   iron
    B   glucose
    C   amino acids
    D   vitamin $B_{12}$
    E   bile salts

*Your answers: A....... B....... C....... D....... E.......*

**30  Vagotomy**

    A   removes the sensation of hunger
    B   decreases gastric acid secretion
    C   produces atrophy of the gastric mucosa
    D   results in doubling of the resting volume of the gall bladder
    E   reduces intestinal motility

*Your answers: A....... B....... C....... D....... E.......*

**31  In the kidney urea**

    A   gives a precise measure of glomerular filtration rate
    B   has a clearance independent of urine flow rate
    C   has a clearance less than that of inulin
    D   is reabsorbed by the renal tubule
    E   is largely responsible for the increased osmolality of the interstitial fluid in the outer medulla

*Your answers: A....... B....... C....... D....... E.......*

**32  In the kidneys the glomeruli**

    A   number about $2.5 \times 10^6$ in total
    B   have afferent arterioles narrower than efferent
    C   have a filtration barrier about $10\,\mu$ thick
    D   have capillary pressures similar to those in the lungs
    E   have active transport mechanisms to control filtrate composition

*Your answers: A....... B....... C....... D....... E.......*

## Practice Exam 4

**33 Reabsorption of sodium in the kidney**

   A   is influenced by hydrostatic pressure and colloid osmotic pressure
   B   occurs in the proximal tubule
   C   is associated with chloride reabsorption
   D   occurs by active transport in the loop of Henle
   E   is regulated by vasopressin

*Your answers: A....... B....... C....... D....... E.......*

**34 The contrast media presently used for X**

   A   usually contain iodine
   B   give better contrast if the person is dehydrated
   C   give better contrast in renal failure
   D   are freely filtered at the glomerulus
   E   are actively secreted in the distal tubule

*Your answers: A....... B....... C....... D....... E.......*

**35 Progesterone**

   A   has a net catabolic effect
   B   is a by-product of androgen degradation
   C   stimulates endometrial secretion
   D   blood concentrations decrease rapidly at term
   E   is not transferred across the placenta to the fetus

*Your answers: A....... B....... C....... D....... E.......*

**36 Graves' disease may be associated with**

   A   thyroidal antibodies
   B   reduced concentrations of TSH
   C   reduced metabolic rate
   D   bradycardia
   E   increased peripheral resistance

*Your answers: A....... B....... C....... D....... E.......*

*Practice Exam 4*

**37 Enhanced growth hormone secretion may be seen**

    A  during starvation
    B  in acromegaly
    C  in gigantism
    D  during exercise
    E  after insulin-induced hypoglycaemia

*Your answers: A....... B....... C....... D....... E.......*

**38 In a nerve an action potential**

    A  has a magnitude dependent on the stimulus strength
    B  is accompanied by hyperpolarisation of the membrane
    C  can potentially travel in either direction
    D  has a velocity which increases with decreased fibre diameter
    E  has a velocity in a peripheral nerve which is reduced with demyelination

*Your answers: A....... B....... C....... D....... E.......*

**39 An excitatory postsynaptic potential (EPSP)**

    A  is produced by acetylcholine liberated from presynaptic endings
    B  represents hyperpolarisation of the postsynaptic membrane
    C  is involved in the activity of motor neurones in the stretch reflex
    D  results in an increase in the permeability of the membrane to sodium, not potassium
    E  may summate with other EPSP's generated in the same cell

*Your answers: A....... B....... C....... D....... E.......*

**40 On complete section of a mixed peripheral nerve**

    A  there is loss of sensation in the denervated area of the skin
    B  the sweat glands in the denervated skin still respond to increases in temperature in the hypothalamus
    C  the temperature of the denervated area will be lower than the affected areas
    D  there is flaccid paralysis
    E  cut fibres lying centrally will not regenerate along the sheath

*Your answers: A....... B....... C....... D....... E.......*

*Practice Exam 4*

**41 Carcinoma of the bladder is associated with**

    A   bladder diverticula
    B   $\beta$ naphthylamine exposure
    C   cigarette smoking
    D   malaria
    E   schistosomiasis

    *Your answers: A....... B....... C....... D....... E.......*

**42 The following are histological types of breast carcinoma**

    A   tubular carcinoma
    B   lobular carcinoma
    C   medullary carcinoma
    D   adenoid cystic carcinoma
    E   duct carcinoma

    *Your answers: A....... B....... C....... D....... E.......*

**43 The following are complications of Cushing's syndrome**

    A   osteomalacia
    B   osteoporosis
    C   osteopetrosis
    D   Kimmelstiel-Wilson lesions
    E   left ventricular hypertrophy

    *Your answers: A....... B....... C....... D....... E.......*

**44 Renal stones may be caused by increased excretion of**

    A   cholesterol
    B   cystine
    C   citrate
    D   urate
    E   xanthine

    *Your answers: A....... B....... C....... D....... E.......*

*Practice Exam 4*

## 45 Avascular necrosis of bone

A may be caused by steroid therapy
B may be caused by irradiation
C may be caused by trauma
D may be caused by prolonged weightlessness
E is another term for a bone infarct

*Your answers:* A....... B....... C....... D....... E.......

## 46 The following statements are true of thiamine

A raw eggs represent a plentiful source
B deficiency causes pellagra
C deficiency may cause heart failure
D deficiency may cause peripheral neuropathy
E may cause an autoimmune haemolytic anaemia

*Your answers:* A....... B....... C....... D....... E.......

## 47 Adult polycystic renal disease

A is inherited as an autosomal dominant condition
B may cause hypertensive heart failure
C may be associated with hepatic and pancreatic cysts
D may be associated with berry aneurysms
E commonly causes microscopic haematuria

*Your answers:* A....... B....... C....... D....... E.......

## 48 The Guthrie test is positive in

A maple syrup disease
B phenylketonuria
C hyperphenylalaninaemia
D Fanconi's syndrome
E galactosaemia

*Your answers:* A....... B....... C....... D....... E.......

*Practice Exam 4*

**49 In sickle cell disease there is/are commonly**

    A  bone marrow hyperplasia
    B  infarction of bone
    C  a decreased serum iron concentration
    D  replacement of glutamic acid by valine in the abnormal haemoglobin
    E  absence of haemoglobin A

*Your answers: A....... B....... C....... D....... E.......*

**50 The following tumours contain neoplastic cells with both epithelial and connective tissue differentiation**

    A  nephroblastoma
    B  neuroblastoma
    C  mixed mesodermal tumour of uterus
    D  teratoma
    E  meningioma

*Your answers: A....... B....... C....... D....... E.......*

**51 Lymph nodes infiltrated by Hodgkin's disease commonly or typically show**

    A  fibrosis
    B  eosinophils
    C  Reed-Sternberg cells
    D  asteroid bodies
    E  abnormal lymph node architecture

*Your answers: A....... B....... C....... D....... E.......*

**52 The following may be of use in the assessment of immunity to diphtheria**

    A  Schick test
    B  Dick test
    C  Frei test
    D  Coomb's test
    E  Kveim test

*Your answers: A....... B....... C....... D....... E.......*

*Practice Exam 4*

**53 Hyperparathyroidism**

  A  may be induced by renal failure
  B  commonly presents as renal stones
  C  is the commonest cause of hypercalcaemia
  D  may cause osteomalacia
  E  is more often due to parathyroid adenoma than parathyroid carcinoma

  *Your answers: A....... B....... C....... D....... E.......*

**54 A female carrier of haemophilia married to a haemophiliac male may produce**

  A  a normal daughter
  B  a normal son
  C  a carrier daughter
  D  a haemophiliac daughter
  E  a haemophiliac son

  *Your answers: A....... B....... C....... D....... E.......*

**55 Examples of active immunisation are**

  A  smallpox vaccination
  B  tetanus toxoid administration
  C  transplacental antibody transfer
  D  BCG injection
  E  antitoxin therapy in diphtheria

  *Your answers: A....... B....... C....... D....... E.......*

**56 In acute lymphoblastic leukaemia**

  A  there is frequently sternal tenderness
  B  chloromas may develop
  C  response to treatment is generally better than in acute myeloid leukaemia
  D  the highest incidence is in the second decade
  E  bleeding manifestations are most appropriately treated with cryoprecipitate

  *Your answers: A....... B....... C....... D....... E.......*

*Practice Exam 4*

**57  In rheumatoid arthritis**

    A   cartilage is the first tissue to be affected
    B   the capsule commonly contains sarcoid-like granulomas
    C   the synovial membrane shows accumulations of lymphocytes and plasma cells
    D   the articular cartilage becomes eroded by pannus
    E   the inflammation causes the cartilage to become fibrillated

    *Your answers: A....... B....... C....... D....... E.......*

**58  Bone marrow failure may develop due to**

    A   miliary tuberculosis
    B   paroxysmal nocturnal haemoglobinuria
    C   therapy with folic acid antagonists
    D   phenylbutazone therapy
    E   Zieve's syndrome

    *Your answers: A....... B....... C....... D....... E.......*

**59  The following tumours commonly arise in bone**

    A   glomus tumour
    B   Ewing's sarcoma
    C   Wilm's tumour
    D   ameloblastoma
    E   myeloid epulis

    *Your answers: A....... B....... C....... D....... E.......*

**60  The following are features of Crohn's disease**

    A   diverticulosis
    B   perforation
    C   more frequent in multiparous than nulliparous women
    D   fistula formation
    E   neuronal hyperplasia

    *Your answers: A....... B....... C....... D....... E.......*

END OF EXAM 4
Go over your answers until your time is up.
Answers and explanations are on page 114.

# PRACTICE EXAM 5

*60 QUESTIONS: Time allowed 2½ hours*

Indicate your answers with a tick or cross in the spaces provided.

1  **The inguinal canal**

   A   is about 6-8 cm long
   B   has the conjoint tendon in its anterior wall
   C   has the ilio-inguinal nerve entering its deep ring
   D   has the inferior epigastric artery medial to its deep ring
   E   has the lacunar (Gimbernat's) ligament in its floor medially

   *Your answers:* A....... B....... C....... D....... E.......

2  **The prostate gland**

   A   is enclosed in a covering of pelvic fascia which is easily separated from its capsule
   B   has lymphatic vessels which go to the sacral nodes
   C   is closely related to the superior facia of the urogenital diaphragm
   D   develops from the urogenital sinus
   E   has veins which are connected to the vertebral venous plexuses

   *Your answers:* A....... B....... C....... D....... E.......

3  **The splanchnic nerves**

   A   are lateral to the ganglionated sympathetic trunk
   B   enter the abdomen by piercing the crura of the diaphragm
   C   contain mainly preganglionic fibres
   D   all end in the coeliac ganglia
   E   are the only source of sympathetic fibres to the abdominal viscera

   *Your answers:* A....... B....... C....... D....... E.......

4  **The pudendal nerve**

   A   passes through the greater sciatic foramen
   B   is medial to the internal pudendal artery on the ischial spine
   C   lies on the medial wall of the ischiorectal fossa
   D   supplies the internal anal sphincter
   E   is sensory to the skin over the symphysis pubis

   *Your answers:* A....... B....... C....... D....... E.......

63

## Practice Exam 5

5  **The ductus arteriosus**

   A  is the only means whereby the blood entering the right atrium bypasses the lungs in the fetus
   B  develops from part of the 4th left aortic arch
   C  is medial to the left recurrent laryngeal nerve
   D  closes at birth due to increased intra-aortic pressure
   E  is closely related to the site of coarctation of the aorta

   *Your answers: A....... B....... C....... D....... E.......*

6  **The pancreas**

   A  is a posterior relation of the stomach
   B  develops from the midgut
   C  has an uncinate process which is posterior to the superior mesenteric vessels
   D  has a head which is anterior to the inferior vena cava
   E  has a body to which is attached the transverse mesocolon

   *Your answers: A....... B....... C....... D....... E.......*

7  **The diaphragm**

   A  is attached to the 1st, 2nd and 3rd lumbar vertebrae by the right crus
   B  has an opening for the inferior vena cava at the level of the 6th thoracic vertebra
   C  has a central tendon which is adherent to the fibrous pericardium
   D  is pierced in its muscular part by the right phrenic nerve
   E  has the sympathetic ganglionated trunk passing behind its lateral arcuate ligament

   *Your answers: A....... B....... C....... D....... E.......*

8  **In the foot**

   A  the superior extensor retinaculum is attached to the tibia and fibula
   B  the dorsalis pedis artery leaves the dorsum through the distal part of the 1st metatarsal space
   C  the tendon of the tibialis anterior muscle is attached to the tuberosity of the navicular
   D  the dorsalis pedis artery is lateral to the tendon of the extensor hallucis longus muscle
   E  the tendon of the peroneus longus muscle is superior to the peroneal trochlea (tubercle)

   *Your answers: A....... B....... C....... D....... E.......*

## Practice Exam 5

**9 At the hip joint**

    A   the capsule is attached posteriorly to the intertrochanteric crest
    B   the ligament of the head of the femur is an important source of blood to the femoral head in the adult
    C   the iliofemoral ligament is attached to the anterior superior iliac spine
    D   the hamstring muscles are supplied by the sciatic nerve
    E   the adductor muscles are supplied by the obturator nerve

*Your answers: A....... B....... C....... D....... E.......*

**10 The ulnar nerve**

    A   in the axilla lies between the axillary artery and vein
    B   is anterior to the medial head of the triceps brachii muscle in the upper arm
    C   is lateral to the ulnar artery in the forearm
    D   enters the hand lateral to the hook of the hamate
    E   gives off its dorsal branch to the hand about 1 cm above the wrist

*Your answers: A....... B....... C....... D....... E.......*

**11 The right vagus nerve in the neck**

    A   supplies the tensor veli palatini (palati) muscle
    B   supplies laryngeal muscles
    C   supplies the sensory side of the cough reflex
    D   supplies the middle constrictor muscle
    E   supplies the stylopharyngeus muscle

*Your answers: A....... B....... C....... D....... E.......*

**12 The posterior triangle (lateral region) of the neck**

    A   has its apex at the inferior nuchal line
    B   has the superior belly of the omohyoid muscle crossing its floor
    C   contains the trunks of the brachial plexus
    D   contains the suprascapular nerve
    E   has the accessory nerve crossing it deep to the prevertebral fascia

*Your answers: A....... B....... C....... D....... E.......*

## Practice Exam 5

### 13 The thymus

A  develops from the endoderm of the foregut
B  develops from the 4th pharyngeal pouch
C  is lobulated in structure
D  decreases in size immediately after birth
E  contains thymic (Hassall's) corpuscles which produce T-lymphocytes

*Your answers: A....... B....... C....... D....... E.......*

### 14 The horizontal (3rd) part of the duodenum

A  is anterior to the abdominal aorta
B  is anterior to the superior mesenteric vessels
C  is at the level of the 1st lumbar vertebra
D  is anterior to the gonadal vessels
E  is posterior to the uncinate process of the pancreas

*Your answers: A....... B....... C....... D....... E.......*

### 15 In the upper arm

A  the thoraco-acromial artery arises lateral to the pectoralis minor muscle
B  the cephalic vein is lateral to the biceps brachii muscle
C  the median nerve crosses anterior to the brachial artery
D  the radial nerve passes anterior to the humerus from the medial to the lateral side
E  the cephalic vein joins the basilic vein to form the axillary vein

*Your answers: A....... B....... C....... D....... E.......*

### 16 The scalenus anterior muscle

A  is posterior to the subclavian vein
B  is posterior to the phrenic nerve
C  medial to the trunks of the brachial plexus
D  is medial to the inferior thyroid artery
E  is medial to the inferior cervical ganglion

*Your answers: A....... B....... C....... D....... E.......*

*Practice Exam 5*

17  The atlas (1st cervical vertebra)

   A  has a small bifid spinous process
   B  has the 1st cervical spinal nerve posterior to the atlanto-occipital joint
   C  has an anterior arch which is larger than its posterior arch
   D  has the rectus capitis posterior major muscle attached to it
   E  has the alar ligaments attached to it

   *Your answers: A....... B....... C....... D....... E.......*

18  With regard to the innervation of the skin of the face and scalp

   A  the mandibular nerve supplies the lower lip
   B  the mandibular nerve supplies part of the lateral side of the scalp
   C  the ophthalmic nerve supplies the lower eyelid
   D  the ventral (anterior primary) ramus of the 1st cervical spinal nerve supplies part of the lateral side of the scalp
   E  the dorsal (posterior primary) rami of the 2nd and 3rd cervical spinal nerves supply the back of the scalp

   *Your answers: A....... B....... C....... D....... E.......*

19  The following are male and female homologous (corresponding) structures

   A  the gubernaculum testis and the ovarian ligament
   B  the ductus (vas) deferens and the round ligament of the uterus
   C  the appendix of the testis and the uterine tube
   D  the bulbo-urethral (Cowper's) glands and the greater vestibular (Bartholin's) glands
   E  the male urethral glands and female urethral glands

   *Your answers: A....... B....... C....... D....... E.......*

20  The vertebral artery

   A  above its origin on the left is posterior to the thoracic duct
   B  has a plexus of preganglionic sympathetic fibres
   C  at the foramen magnum is posterior to the spinal accessory nerve
   D  supplies the spinal cord
   E  supplies the cerebellum

   *Your answers: A....... B....... C....... D....... E.......*

*Practice Exam 5*

## 21 Vasoconstriction follows

   A   the Valsalva manoeuvre
   B   asphyxia
   C   lying down
   D   carotid occlusion
   E   blood loss

*Your answers: A....... B....... C....... D....... E.......*

## 22 The result of stimulation of the sympathetic nerves to the heart

   A   is increased oxygen consumption by the heart
   B   increased cardiac output
   C   increased coronary blood flow
   D   a shift to the right of the plot of myocardial contractility versus fibre length
   E   an increase in the slope of the pacemaker potential in the sinoatrial cells

*Your answers: A....... B....... C....... D....... E.......*

## 23 Carbon dioxide may be transported

   A   at a partial pressure of 6kPa (46 mm Hg) in arterial blood
   B   largely as bicarbonate in the erythrocytes
   C   as a carbamino compound with haemoglobin
   D   in association with plasma protein
   E   physically dissolved

*Your answers: A....... B....... C....... D....... E.......*

## 24 During the cardiac cycle

   A   the second heart sound is caused by closure of the aortic and pulmonary valves
   B   the period of rapid ventricular filling occurs in early diastole
   C   the pressure in diastole is higher in the aorta than in the left ventricle
   D   in mid-diastole the pressure in the right atrium is slightly higher than in the right ventricle
   E   the thin walled atria merely act as venous reservoirs

*Your answers: A....... B....... C....... D....... E.......*

*Practice Exam 5*

**25 The respiratory centre in the brain stem**

   A  comprises anatomically distinct inspiratory and expiratory centres
   B  has inherent rhythmicity
   C  is unaffected by shifts in blood hydrogen ion concentration
   D  may be influenced by pain
   E  can be influenced by inputs from the limbic system and hypothalamus

*Your answers: A....... B....... C....... D....... E.......*

**26 Decreased arterial oxygen tension can result from**

   A  abnormal matching of ventilation and blood flow
   B  decreased airway resistance
   C  ascent to high altitude
   D  low haemoglobin concentration
   E  carbon monoxide poisoning

*Your answers: A....... B....... C....... D....... E.......*

**27 Rapid ways of reducing plasma potassium include**

   A  dialysis of the patient
   B  administration of a potassium free diet
   C  administration of chlorpropamide
   D  infusion of hypertonic sodium chloride
   E  infusion of glucose and insulin

*Your answers: A....... B....... C....... D....... E.......*

**28 Intrinsic factor**

   A  is found in the liver
   B  is found in the terminal ileum
   C  is produced in parietal cells
   D  aids absorption of folic acid
   E  deficiency can be treated with injections of $B_{12}$

*Your answers: A....... B....... C....... D....... E.......*

*Practice Exam 5*

### 29 Active transport

A uses energy derived solely from anaerobic processes
B is increased by hypothermia
C prevents cells from swelling
D is one of the mechanisms for absorption of glucose in the small intestine
E is involved in hydrogen ion secretion by the kidney tubule cells

*Your answers: A....... B....... C....... D....... E.......*

### 30 In megacolon

A the ganglia of the intrinsic plexuses degenerate
B the proximal part of the colon becomes grossly distended
C diarrhoea is quite common
D peristaltic movement is greatly increased
E a large proportion of water reabsorption may occur in the colon

*Your answers: A....... B....... C....... D....... E.......*

### 31 If a healthy person has no food for a week

A blood glucose is likely to fall below 2.5 mmol/1 (50mg%)
B glucose is formed in the liver from amino acids
C insulin secretion decreases
D the brain metabolises free fatty acids
E the muscles metabolise free fatty acids

*Your answers: A....... B....... C....... D....... E.......*

### 32 Oedema can occur as a result of

A liver disease
B vasodilatation
C an increase in plasma albumin
D obstruction of the lymphatic vessels
E increase in the capillary pressure to 37 mmHg

*Your answers: A....... B....... C....... D....... E.......*

Practice Exam 5

33 **In the proximal tubule**

   A  the fluid is hypotonic
   B  the major force for filtrate reabsorption is active absorption of chloride
   C  sodium transport is controlled by aldosterone
   D  PAH is actively secreted
   E  hydrogen ion is secreted

   *Your answers: A....... B....... C....... D....... E.......*

34 **In the case of fully compensated respiratory acidosis**

   A  arterial $pCO_2$ is raised
   B  plasma pH is reduced
   C  there is reduced plasma bicarbonate
   D  there is an abnormal bicarbonate: $pCO_2$ ratio in plasma
   E  base excess is normal

   *Your answers: A....... B....... C....... D....... E.......*

35 **The hormones secreted by the anterior pituitary include**

   A  somatostatin
   B  prolactin
   C  oxytocin
   D  aldosterone
   E  thyrotrophin

   *Your answers: A....... B....... C....... D....... E.......*

36 **Over the course of the normal menstrual cycle**

   A  oestradiol secretion increases over the first 14 days
   B  the endometrium proliferates over the first 14 days
   C  the cervical mucous secretion is thinner mid-cycle
   D  body temperature decreases mid-cycle
   E  over days 14-28 the endometrium secretes gonadotrophins

   *Your answers: A....... B....... C....... D....... E.......*

*Practice Exam 5*

37  **A low plasma calcium**

    A   is one of less than 5.0 mM
    B   is associated with vitamin D deficiency
    C   results in hyperexcitability of peripheral nerves
    D   is associated with increased calcitonin release
    E   is associated with increased plasma phosphate

    *Your answers:* A....... B....... C....... D....... E.......

38  **Glucagon**

    A   is produced by the pancreatic $\beta$ cells
    B   is a polypeptide hormone
    C   secretion is stimulated during fasting
    D   inhibits insulin production
    E   stimulates liver phosphorylation

    *Your answers:* A....... B....... C....... D....... E.......

39  **Paralysis of the sympathetic nerve supply to the head could lead to**

    A   lack of sweating over the face
    B   arteriolar vasoconstriction
    C   ptosis (drooping of the eyelid)
    D   miosis (constriction of the pupil)
    E   inability of the eye to accommodate

    *Your answers:* A....... B....... C....... D....... E.......

40  **If one pours cold water (30° C) into the external auditory meatus of a supine subject with their head tilted forward (caloric testing)**

    A   vestibulo-ocular reflexes occur in an unconscious subject providing the brain stem is functioning
    B   the convection currents produced cause nystagmus
    C   nystagmus will not occur for 20 seconds
    D   the quick phase of nystagmus is towards the cooled side
    E   the duration of nystagmus may be used for diagnosis of damage to the vestibular apparatus and the nervous connections

    *Your answers:* A....... B....... C....... D....... E.......

*Practice Exam 5*

**41 A malignant tumour is the usual cause of**

    A    Conn's syndrome
    B    acromegaly
    C    Cushing's syndrome
    D    paroxysmal hypertension
    E    hyperparathyroidism

*Your answers: A....... B....... C....... D....... E.......*

**42 Myocardial infarction may be complicated by**

    A    cardiac aneurysm
    B    giant cell myocarditis
    C    focal glomerulonephritis
    D    dissecting aneurysm of aorta
    E    cerebral infarction

*Your answers: A....... B....... C....... D....... E.......*

**43 Molluscum sebaceum**

    A    is an alternative name for keratoacanthoma
    B    is a premalignant condition
    C    is a variety of sebaceous cyst
    D    is caused by a virus of the pox group
    E    may remit spontaneously

*Your answers: A....... B....... C....... D....... E.......*

**44 Metastatic calcification is seen in**

    A    hyperparathyroidism
    B    sarcoidosis
    C    fat necrosis
    D    atheroma
    E    myositis ossificans

*Your answers: A....... B....... C....... D....... E.......*

*Practice Exam 5*

**45  Barr bodies may be found in the neutrophils of**

    A   normal females
    B   normal males
    C   male patients with chronic granulocytic leukaemia
    D   patients with Klinefelter's syndrome
    E   patients with Turner's syndrome

*Your answers: A....... B....... C....... D....... E.......*

**46  There is a predisposition towards left ventricular failure with**

    A   aortic stenosis
    B   mitral stenosis
    C   mitral incompetence
    D   pulmonary hypertension
    E   atrial septal defect

*Your answers: A....... B....... C....... D....... E.......*

**47  The following are features of diabetic ketosis**

    A   high body potassium content
    B   decreased blood hydrogen ion activity
    C   water depletion
    D   high plasma total carbon dioxide
    E   hyperkalaemia

*Your answers: A....... B....... C....... D....... E.......*

**48  The following individuals carry at least one abnormal gene**

    A   father of colour-blind girl
    B   mother of child with cystic fibrosis
    C   father of haemophiliac boy
    D   haemophiliac boy
    E   mother of a child with familial polyposis

*Your answers: A....... B....... C....... D....... E.......*

## Practice Exam 5

**49 Pernicious anaemia**

 A  is sometimes one of the results of the malabsorption syndrome
 B  can be caused by tape worm infestation
 C  may cause thrombocytopenia
 D  causes a peripheral neuropathy
 E  is associated with carcinoma of the stomach

*Your answers: A....... B....... C....... D....... E.......*

**50 The following neoplasms occur more commonly in children than in adults**

 A  meningioma
 B  medulloblastoma
 C  carcinoid tumour of appendix
 D  chondrosarcoma
 E  teratoma

*Your answers: A....... B....... C....... D....... E.......*

**51 The reticulocyte count is raised**

 A  in severe iron deficiency anaemia
 B  following haemorrhage
 C  after a lethal dose of radiation
 D  in patients with polycythaemia rubra vera
 E  soon after $B_{12}$ administration to patients with pernicious anaemia

*Your answers: A....... B....... C....... D....... E.......*

**52 The following are typical of chronic myeloid leukaemia**

 A  deletion of chromosome 9
 B  splenomegaly
 C  frequent in childhood
 D  hyperplastic marrow
 E  raised neutrophil alkaline phosphatase

*Your answers: A....... B....... C....... D....... E.......*

## Practice Exam 5

**53 Amyloidosis is a recognised complication of**

A Hodgkin's disease
B papillary carcinoma of thyroid
C pernicious anaemia
D rheumatoid arthritis
E Crohn's disease

Your answers: A....... B....... C....... D....... E.......

**54 The normal range of a serum component is generally defined by**

A mean ± one standard deviation
B mean ± two standard deviations
C mean ± three standard deviations
D limits excluding the upper and lower 2.5% of a normal population
E limits excluding the upper and lower 5% of a normal population

Your answers: A....... B....... C....... D....... E.......

**55 Rickettsiae**

A are primarily intestinal parasites of insects
B contain both RNA and DNA
C are generally gram positive
D are sensitive to tetracycline
E grow in the yolk sac of chick embryos

Your answers: A....... B....... C....... D....... E.......

**56 The following organisms may cause food poisoning**

A *Staphylococcus aureus*
B *Staphylococcus albus*
C *Clostridium tetani*
D *Clostridium welchii*
E *Clostridium botulinum*

Your answers: A....... B....... C....... D....... E.......

*Practice Exam 5*

**57  Ankylostoma**

    A   embryos enter through the skin
    B   may cause an unproductive cough
    C   uses dogs as intermediate hosts
    D   can cause intestinal ulceration
    E   infestation is common in subtropical countries

*Your answers: A....... B....... C....... D....... E.......*

**58  Immunisation against *Mycobacterium tuberculosis* is most successful using**

    A   PPD
    B   formalin-killed organisms
    C   live attenuated organisms
    D   tuberculin
    E   specific antiserum

*Your answers: A....... B....... C....... D....... E.......*

**59  In osteoarthritis there is commonly**

    A   osteophyte formation
    B   lymphoid follicle formation in the synovium
    C   raised alkaline phosphatase
    D   low serum calcium
    E   fibrillation of joint cartilage

*Your answers: A....... B....... C....... D....... E.......*

**60  The following conditions are associated with an increased incidence of cutaneous malignancy**

    A   acanthosis nigricans
    B   leukoplakia
    C   solar keratosis
    D   Bowen's disease
    E   squamous papilloma

*Your answers: A....... B....... C....... D....... E.......*

END OF EXAM 5
Go over your answers until your time is up.
Answers and explanations are on page 126.

# ANSWERS AND EXPLANATIONS

## ANSWERS TO PRACTICE EXAM 1

The correct answer options are given against each question.

1 **A B**

Normally a child has all its deciduous teeth by about 2 years of age. There are 5 in each quadrant. The lingual nerve lies in a groove just below the crown of the 3rd molar in an adult, or the 2nd molar in a child before the 3rd molar erupts. The mandible ossifies in membrane round Meckel's cartilage which is in the 1st arch and together with other areas of cartilage (head of mandible, coronoid process, symphysis menti) is invaded by bone. There is an articular disc between the head of the mandible and the temporal bone in the temporomandibular joint.

2 **A C**

In the new terminology the left coronary artery is a short artery. It passes forwards and divides into the anterior interventricular and circumflex arteries. The circumflex continues in the coronary sulcus. All investigations have shown that there are anastomoses between the two coronary arteries although they are usually described as 'end-arteries'. A better term would be 'functional end-arteries' because following a sudden blocking of a coronary artery or one of the large branches no effective anastomosis takes place. The posterior interventricular branch comes from the right coronary artery. The atrioventricular node is supplied by the right coronary artery in more than 80% of hearts.

3 **D E**

The long thoracic nerve arises from the roots (the ventral rami of C5, 6, 7), the suprascapular nerve from the upper trunk (C5,6) and the musculocutaneous nerve (C5, 6, 7) from the lateral cord. There are three branches (the two subscapular and thoracodorsal nerves) from the posterior cord before it divides into its two terminal branches (the radial and axillary nerves). The three branches supply the three muscles of the posterior axillary wall.

4 **A E**

The stomach, a derivative of the foregut, is supplied by branches of the coeliac artery, or their branches. The short gastric arteries lie in the gastrosplenic not the lienorenal ligament. The right gastric artery is from the hepatic artery as a rule, the left gastric artery comes from the coeliac, and both run along the lesser curvature. The gastro-epiploic arteries (right from the gastroduodenal, left from the splenic) run along the greater curvature.

*Answers and Explanations Practice Exam 1*

**5 E**

The external anal sphincter and anus form the medial wall of the ischiorectal fossa inferior to the levator ani, below the level of the rectum. There is considerable confusion in the terminology related to the anal canal and rectum, for example, their blood and nerve supply, and the term 'rectal examination'. There is peritoneum on the front of and sides of the upper third and the front of the middle third of the rectum. The lower third is below the level of the peritoneum which passes forwards towards the uterus or bladder. The rectum has neither appendices epiploicae nor taeniae coli which are characteristic of most of the large intestine.

**6 C D**

The oesophagus begins at the level of the 6th cervical vertebra (and the cricoid cartilage). It is narrowed by the left bronchus because the trachea divides a little to the right of the midline. It is usually constricted at its commencement, by the arch of the aorta and where it passes through the diaphragm. Beyond the trachea the oesophagus lies behind the heart (the left atrium) separated by the pericardium. The beginning of the oesophagus is about 15 cm from the incisor teeth, the level of the left bronchus is about 25 cm from the incisor teeth and the level of the diaphragm is about 40 cm from the incisor teeth. The thoracic duct runs upwards behind the right border of the oesophagus to about the level of the 5th thoracic vertebra then crosses to the left behind the oesophagus and continues upwards behind its left border.

**7 A C D**

It is generally agreed that although sympathetic nerves cause vasoconstriction, they are vasodilator to the coronary arteries and the vessels of skeletal muscle. Parasympathetic fibres cause the smooth muscle of the bronchial tree to contract. Grey rami communicantes are postganglionic sympathetic fibres and are almost all adrenergic. The sweat gland innervation is an exception. The sphincter pupillae and ciliary muscle are supplied by postganglionic parasympathetic fibres and the dilatator pupillae by the sympathetic.

*Answers and Explanations Practice Exam 1*

**8 A D**
The neck of the gall bladder is anterior to the superior part of the duodenum and its body is anterior to the transverse colon. Although the origin of the cystic artery is very variable it most commonly is a branch of the right hepatic artery. The cystic vein usually goes to the portal vein. Other acceptable surface markings for the fundus are 1) where the midclavicular line crosses the costal margin 2) where the transpyloric plane crosses the costal margin. The tip of the 9th costal cartilage is difficult to find. The colummnar epithelium lining the gall bladder has few if any goblet cells.

**9 A B C**
The brachial artery usually divides into the radial and ulnar arteries at the level of the neck of the radius. The ulnar artery then passes deep to the pronator teres muscle and the flexor digitorum superficialis muscles. It then lies lateral to the ulnar nerve on the flexor digitorum profundus muscle overlapped by the flexor carpi radialis muscle. At the wrist it enters the hand superficial to the flexor retinaculum lateral to the pisiform bone. In about 2% of people the ulnar artery may be superficial and must not be mistakaen for a vein (note that it pulsates, unlike a vein).

**10 A B C**
The shafts of the metacarpals and phalanges begin to ossify between the 8th and 12th weeks of fetal life (distal phalanx, metacarpal, proximal phalanx and middle phalanx, in that order). As a rule, all the carpal bones are cartilaginous at birth. They ossify in what is described as a spiral order beginning with the capitate (2nd month after birth), then the hamate (3rd month after birth), triquetral (3rd year), lunate (4th year), scaphoid, trapezium and trapezoid (5th year). The pisiform does not ossify until the 9th or 10th year in females and the 11th year in males. In the female, ossification including fusion of epiphyses occurs earlier than in the male, a difference of weeks in the fetus, and months or years after birth.

## Answers and Explanations Practice Exam 1

**11 A B C E**
The hypoglossal canal (anterior condyloid foramen) in the occipital bone is medial to the jugular foramen. The hypoglossal nerve lies inferior to the lingual nerve on the superficial surface of the hyoglossus muscle together with the deep part of the submandibular gland and its duct and the submandibular ganglion. The lingual artery loops upwards on the middle constrictor muscle of the pharynx and is crossed superficially by the hypoglossal nerve. The palatoglossus muscle is supplied by the pharyngeal plexus of nerves, the motor branch of which is the pharyngeal branch of the vagus.

**12 B C D E**
The ischiocavernosus muscle covers the crus of the penis or clitoris as it lies along the ischiopubic ramus. The bulbospongiosus muscle lies round the bulb of the penis in the midline or the bulbs of the vestibule around the vagina, and posteriorly is attached to the perineal body. The levatores ani pass downwards and medially from their lateral attachments and meet in the midline except where they surround the midline viscera. Other muscles contributing fibres to the perineal body are the transverse perineal muscles, the deep and superficial parts of the external anal sphincter and the sphincter urethrae.

**13 C D**
The ophthalmic artery enters the orbit through the optic canal and its branches supply all three coats. The lacrimal gland is in two parts, an orbital above the levator and a palpebral below it. The two parts are joined round the lateral border or the aponeurosis of the muscle. The inferior ophthalmic vein may join the superior which always goes to the cavernous sinus. The absence of valves allows blood to flow in both directions.

**14 B C**
The flexor pollicis longus is not paralysed - it is supplied by the anterior interosseous nerve, a branch of the median, in the fore-arm. The opponens pollicis is paralysed because it is supplied in the palm by a branch of the median nerve. The digital branches of the median nerve supply the skin dorsal to the terminal phalanx and the nail bed. The skin on the lateral side of the palm is supplied by the palmar branch of the median nerve which is given off in the lower part of the forearm. The abductor pollicis longus is supplied by the radial nerve.

## Answers and Explanations Practice Exam 1

**15 A C D**
The pterygopalatine ganglion in the pterygopalatine fossa receives the nerve of the pterygoid canal which contains both sympathetic and parasympathetic fibres. The postganglionic fibres supply the lacrimal gland and also the glands of the palate and nasal cavity. The white rami communicantes from the intercostal nerves to the thoracic part of the sympathetic trunk are preganglionic. The grey rami communicantes are postganglionic and leave the sympathetic trunk at all levels. The pelvic plexuses are both sympathetic, from the superior hypogastric plexus (the presacral nerve) and grey rami communicantes from the sacral sympathetic ganglia, and parasympathetic from S2, 3, 4, the pelvic splanchnic nerves. The vagus nerve is mainly preganglionic parasympathetic.

**16 A C D**
The floor of the inguinal canal along its whole length is formed by the inguinal ligament. The lacunar ligament is in its floor medially. The posterior wall along its whole length is formed by the fascia transversalis which is strengthened medially by the conjoint tendon formed by the lowest fibres of the internal oblique and transversus abdominis muscles arching over the canal medially. Fibres from the internal oblique thus form a roof to the canal. The round ligament of the uterus passes through the inguinal canal and goes into the labium majus. The ligament is the remains of the gubernaculum ovarii.

**17 A C E**
More accurately, the lateral boundary of the femoral triangle is formed by the medial border of the sartorius muscle and the medial boundary by the medial border of the adductor longus; the inguinal ligament forms the 3rd side. The muscles in the floor are the iliopsoas, pectineus and adductor longus. The femoral nerve is lateral to and outside the femoral sheath which contains the femoral artery and vein and femoral canal. The triangle is roofed over by the fascia lata in which there is the saphenous opening for the great saphenous vein.

**18 A B C D**
The pia mater is the layer which forms the ligamenta denticulata. These tooth-like lateral projections help anchor the spinal cord within the vertebral canal.

*Answers and Explanations Practice Exam 1*

**19 B D**
The pleuroperitoneal canals usually close by the 9th week. The distal parts of the paramesonephric ducts have fused by the 10th week. The distal parts of the paramesonephric ducts have fused by the 10th week. The testes do not enter the inguinal canal until about the 25th week. The so-called umbilical midgut hernia is present from the 6th to the 12th weeks. Haemopoiesis takes place mainly in the red bone marrow by the 12th week.

**20 A B E**
The first posterior intercostal vein on both sides goes to either the brachiocephalic vein or the vertebral vein. The second and third veins form the superior intercostal vein. On the right, it goes to the azygos vein, on the left to the left brachiocephalic. The rest of the right posterior intercostal veins join the azygos vein. The upper left posterior intercostal veins form the accessory hemiazygos vein and the lower form the hemiazygos vein (former names were superior and inferior hemiazygos veins). Both horizontal structures are external to the vertical structures.

**21 C**
Severe burns produce a fall in plasma volume producing hypovolaemic shock similar to that of haemorrhage. The characteristics of the two conditions are similar but with burns the blood viscosity can increase as a result of the loss of plasma and this exacerbates the sluggishness of the blood flow.

**22 B C E**
As for flow of fluid or electrical current, $R = P/Q$, where R is the resistance to flow, P is the pressure gradient across the tube and Q is the volume flow rate. Poiseuille, a French physician, observed that the volume flow rate through a tube was affected by the pressure difference between the ends of the tube, the viscosity of the fluid and the tube radius and length. Poiseuille's equation may be rewritten to give $P/Q = R = 8\eta l/r^4$ where $\eta$ is the viscosity of the blood, which depends on the haematocrit, and r is the radius of the blood vessel and l the length.

**23 B C D E**
The mean systemic filling pressure is the pressure measured in the systemic vessels when the root of the aorta and great veins entering the heart have suddenly been clamped and all the pressures in the systemic system are brought to instant equilibrium. Three main factors are found to change it; blood volume changes, alteration in the sympathetic tone and skeletal muscle contraction.

## Answers and Explanations Practice Exam 1

**24 B C D E**
Irritant receptors are located in the epithelium of large predominantly extrapulmonary airways. They can be stimulated both by inhalation of irritant material or mechanically, resulting in hyperpnoea, bronchoconstriction and often coughing. Irritant reflex information is transmitted via myelinated vagal afferents.

**25 A B C E**
Oxygen at high tensions produces a small increase in oxygen saturation in the blood leading to a small fall in pulmonary ventilation, but not apnoea. Oxygen at high pressure has a number of toxic properties, producing vasoconstriction of the cerebral vessels and brain damage; also nausea and muscle twitching. Hyperbaric oxygen drives off carbon monoxide from blood more rapidly than normal.

**26 B C D**
The magnitude of the change in lung volume (V) caused by a given change in the pressure difference across the lung wall ($\delta$) is defined as lung compliance. It is measured under static conditions. Increased lung recoil as in pulmonary fibrosis causes a low compliance. Decreasing recoil as in emphysema leads to high compliance.

**27 A B C D**
Metabolic activity can be increased markedly by increased muscle activity, either exercise or shivering. The hormones able to produce an increase in metabolic activity of up to 40% are catecholamines and the thyroid hormones. Insulin has no such effect.

**28 B D**
Blood buffers form part of an integrated system. The two main buffers in blood are bicarbonate and haemoglobin, although the sodium salts of phosphate and plasma proteins also contribute. Ammonium ions are important in buffering hydrogen ions in the urine.

**29 A D**
Very intense irritation of the intestinal mucosa, as occurs in some infective processes, can elicit a peristaltic rush which is a powerful peristaltic wave that travels long distances in the small intestine. In a few minutes waves can sweep the contents of the intestine into the colon and thereby relieve the small intestine of either irritative chyme or excessive distension.

*Answers and Explanations Practice Exam 1*

**30 B**
Hunger contractions are usually rhythmic peristaltic contractions probably representing exacerbated mixing waves in the body of the stomach. However, when they become extremely strong, they often fuse together and can cause tetanic contractions as long as 2 - 3 minutes. They are most intense in young healthy individuals and are increased by low blood sugar. They do not begin until 12 - 24 hours after food was last ingested and reach their greatest intensity in 3 - 4 days and then subside.

**31 A C E**
The Zollinger-Ellison syndrome is caused by a pancreatic tumour, secreting large amounts of gastrin with a resultant increase in basal gastrin secretion. It is characterised by recurrent peptic ulcers. Injections of secretin release gastrin from the tumour.

**32 B C D E**
A concentration gradient exists across the kidney which is produced by the counter-current multiplier system. It depends on the active transport of chloride from the thick ascending limb which is impermeable to water. The water leaves by the thick descending limb which is permeable to water. As the process depends on active transport, the gradient is dissipated at $0°C$.

**33 C D E**
In secondary dehydration there is a loss of salt in excess of water so that the osmolality of the extracellular fluid decreases and fluid tends to enter the cells. This results in reduced secretion of antidiuretic hormone so that a good flow of dilute urine is maintained. Fluid is lost from the extracellular compartment so that plasma protein concentration and packed cell volume is increased.

**34 A B D E**
Substances that are filtered by the glomerulus, but not reabsorbed, or whose quantities filtered exceed the reabsorptive capacity of the cells of the nephron, may retard absorption of salt and water by their osmotic effects. In sufficient quantities mannitol and glucose are such substances.

**35 B C D E**
The alkalosis, renal features, polyuria and nocturia and the muscular ones of weakness are due to hypokalaemia. Other features of over-production of aldosterone are hypertensive vascular disease.

*Answers and Explanations Practice Exam 1*

**36 B C E**
Insulin is the main form of therapy in ketonic diabetes. The requirements may be reduced by exercise and weight reduction. In general management of diabetes mellitus involves several inter-related approaches including diet and oral hypoglycaemics such as chlorpropamide. Control of diet is not necessarily the best way to manage glycosuria or to prevent arteriosclerosis.

**37 A B C**
Alteration in the binding capacity of thyroid-binding globulin is increased by many diseases and drugs as well as genetic defects. There is increased binding capacity during pregnancy and following oestrogen treatment (including the contraceptive pill). It is also increased in myxoedema. In general, alterations of thyroid binding capacity do not affect thyroid status.

**38 A E**
The control of prolactin secretion is unusal in that its release is tonically inhibited by the hypothalamus via the action of PIF. There is evidence that prolactin release is inhibited by increased plasma prolactin levels (shortloop feed-back). The hypothalamic hormone TRH will stimulate prolactin release, not inhibit it. Neither oxytocin nor somatostatin are thought to inhibit prolactin release.

**39 A B D E**
The cerebellum is chiefly involved in skeletal muscle movement. It helps provide smooth directed movements and to maintain balance. It is not involved in the initiation of movement.

**40 A C E**
The cutaneous receptors in the free nerve endings, Ruffini's endings and Pacinian corpuscles all respond to mechanical deformation. The carotid baroreceptors, sensitive to changes in blood pressure, respond to stretch. Schwann cells are not nerve endings, but are associated with nerve fibres.

**41 A C E**
Malaria causes haemolysis by parasitic destruction of red cells and by hypersplenism. Haemolysis is caused by G6PD deficiency in which the haemoglobin is less well protected against oxidation. Abnormal haemoglobins, such as sickle cell haemoglobin, render cells more prone to haemolysis.

**42 C E**
Schaumann bodies are spherical basophilic masses seen in macrophage giant cells. They are particularly common in sarcoidosis, but are also seen in many other granulomatous disorders.

**43 B E**
Osteosarcomas and giant cell tumours (osteoclastomas) are primary neoplasms (autonomous new growths) of bone.

**44 A C E**
Magnesium deficiency may cause tetany, correctable by magnesium but not by calcium. Reduced absorption (malabsorption) or intake (alcoholics) causes the plasma concentration to fall. Magnesium is normally excreted by the kidneys, and it therefore accumulates in chronic renal failure.

**45 A B C D E**
Bacteroides are frequently involved in infections of tissues with low oxygen tension, in septic abortions, post partum uterine infections, and in pus from intra-abdominal lesions, cerebral, dental and soft tissue abscesses. They usually cause infection in association with other anaerobes, or aerobic organisms, notably *E.coli*, when synergy may be responsible for most of the tissue damage.

**46 A B C E**
*Pseudomonas aeruginosa* is a strict aerobe commonly found in the human intestine, which has the ability to survive and grow in almost any moist situation, even in weak disinfectant solutions, over a wide temperature range.

**47 B D E**
Alpha-fetoprotein is raised in most cases of hepatoma and testicular teratoma, and often in hepatitis and colitis. A raised alpha-fetoprotein is found in amniotic fluid and in maternal serum when there is a fetal neural tube defect. Carcinoembryonic antigen is often raised in neuroblastoma and carcinoma of colon and pancreas.

**48 B C E**
Basophil adenomas cause Cushing's syndrome, acidophil adenomas cause acromegaly. Pressure atrophy of the remainder of the pituitary may cause hypothyroidism and amenorrhoea. Craniopharyngiomas arise from the craniopharyngeal duct remnants.

## Answers and Explanations Practice Exam 1

**49 B**
Individuals of blood group A constitutionally possess anti B antibodies, but only produce antibodies to rhesus groups (C, D, E) after transfusion with rhesus positive blood.

**50 A D E**
Polycythemia is a response to chronic hypoxia, one cause of which is right-to-left shunts. It is sometimes seen in adenocarcinoma of the kidney and in Cushing's syndrome.

**51 B**
Purine synthesis is increased in primary hyperuricaemia. Some patients also have a reduced urate secretion. Debauchery and intemperence may precipitate gout in patients with the underlying biochemical lesion, by causing increased intake of purines (high protein diet) and alcoholism predisposes to the development of gout, perhaps by producing lactic acidaemia.

**52 B C E**
Haemachromatosis, a congenital disease associated with increased iron absorption, causes iron accumulation in many types of parenchymal cells throughout the body, including hepatocytes. In haemosiderosis iron accumulates in the reticulo-endothelial system, and parenchymal cells are little affected. Paroxysmal nocturnal haemoglobinuria is one cause of hepatic vein thrombosis (Budd-Chiari syndrome).

**53 B D**
Syphilis causes saccular or fusiform aneurysms of the thoracic aorta. The inflammatory process causes endarteritis of vasa vasorum and causes fibrous replacement of the aortic media, and allows stretching of the aortic value ring. Syphilis is characterised by accumulations of plasma cells.

**54 B E**
Although cytomegalovirus can cause a similar disease in which atypical mononuclear cells are present in the blood, infectious mononucleosis is caused by the Epstein-Barr virus. Lymphocytosis is the rule, and many of these are atypical when inspected in a blood film. Anaemia is unusual but may be caused by haemolysis. The serum contains antibodies which agglutinate sheep red cells unless first absorbed by ox cells.

## Answers and Explanations Practice Exam 1

**55 A B**
The intracerebral haemorrhage which is a complication of untreated benign hypertension is associated with the presence of microaneurysms of intracerebral arteries. Middle meningeal arterial haemorrhage is extradural.

**56 C D**
In Fallot's tetralogy there is right ventricular hypertrophy. In coarctation of the aorta there is narrowing of the aorta at the site of the ductus arteriosus, and increased blood pressure compensates for reduced flow.

**57 D**
If tumour is confined within the bowel wall it is stage A; if it has reached serosa it is B. If lymph node metastases are present it is stage C irrespective of the extent of local spread. Staging is performed on a macroscopic and microscopic appearance of the surgically resected specimen and thus cannot involve an assessment of distant metastases.

**58 B C D E**
Atheroma is associated with congenital or acquired increase in serum low density lipoprotein levels; increased high density lipoproteins are associated with reduced atheroma. Pulmonary hypertension causes atheroma in pulmonary arteries.

**59 A E**
*Actinomyces israelii* is a gram-positive anaerobe. Standard treatment is high-dose penicillin. It spreads by blood and by contiguous spread. Intrauterine contraceptive devices predispose to pelvic actinomycosis. It is a large bowel commensal; abdominal actinomycosis may follow appendicitis.

**60 B D E**
Polymorphs are unable to multiply. They are actively motile and phagocytic, and the granules seen in the light microscope are lysosomes. Only lymphoid cells are able to produce immunoglobulin.

# ANSWERS TO PRACTICE EXAM 2

**1  C D E**
The radial nerve (superficial branch) leaves the radial artery well above the wrist and passes backwards deep to the brachioradialis muscle. The radial artery is deep to the tendon of the extensor pollicis longus and then enters the palm between the heads of the first dorsal interosseous muscle to form the deep palmar arch. Its dorsal carpal branch gives off metacarpal branches which in turn give off digital branches. The radial artery in the palm gives off two large branches, one to the thumb and one to the index finger.

**2  A C D**
The midgut extends from the middle of the descending (2nd) part of the duodenum, distal to the opening of the bile and pancreatic ducts, to the junction of the right two-thirds and left one-third of the transverse colon. Meckel's (ileal) diverticulum is the remains of a persistent vitello-intestinal duct which connects the gut to the yolk sac from which most of the alimentary tract and its derivatives (liver, pancreas) develop.

**3  B D**
The anterior wall of the axilla is in two layers, a superficial formed by the pectoralis major muscle and a deep by the clavicle, subclavius muscle, clavipectoral fascia and pectoralis minor. The posterior wall is formed by the subscapularis, latissimus dorsi and teres major muscles. The medial wall is formed by the upper ribs and the serratus anterior muscle and the lateral wall by the shaft of the humerus and the coracobrachialis muscle. The long thoracic nerve supplies the serratus anterior and descends on its superficial surface. The roots and trunks of the brachial plexus are in the neck above the clavicle, its divisions are behind the clavicle and its cords with their branches are below the clavicle in the axilla itself.

**4  B D E**
The hypothalamus is part of the forebrain, forms part of the floor of the 3rd ventricle, and is usually said to extend externally from the optic chiasma to the mamillary bodies, with the tuber cinereum between these structures. The infundibulum (stalk) of the hypophysis cerebri (pituitary gland) is attached to the tuber cinereum. The vasopressin of the posterior lobe of the pituitary is formed in the hypothalamus. The lamina terminalis, the original rostral end of the neural tube, extends upwards from the optic chiasma to the anterior commissure in front of the optic nuclei of the hypothalamus related to the optic chiasma.

## Answers and Explanations Practice Exam 2

**5  A B E**
The basilic vein at the elbow is the only vein in this region which has cutaneous nerve branches superficial to it. It becomes deep about the middle of the upper arm and joins the brachial veins to form the axillary vein. The cephalic vein, on the lateral side of the upper limb, becomes deep between the deltoid and pectoralis major muscles and joins the axillary vein just proximal to the clavicle.

**6  A C D**
The superior rectus muscle acts with the inferior oblique muscle (pulls the eyeball upwards and outwards) to pull the eyeball upwards. The superior oblique muscle hooks round the trochlea (pulley) in the anterior superior medial corner of the orbit and passes laterally and backwards so that it pulls the eyeball downwards and outwards. The central artery of the retina is a branch of the ophthalmic artery and at first is inferior to the optic nerve. About 1 cm behind the eyeball the artery sinks into the substance of the nerve. The levator palpebrae superioris contains both striated and smooth muscle and is supplied by the oculomotor nerve and postganglionic sympathetic fibres. The optic nerve develops as an outgrowth from the forebrain and takes with it the three meninges.

**7  A C D E**
The phrenic nerve from the 3rd, 4th and 5th cervical spinal nerves is both motor and sensory. The lower intercostal nerves which supply the periphery of the diaphragm are sensory. When paralysed, for example, after a 'phrenic crush', one half of the diaphragm rises towards the thoracic cavity. When the diaphragm contracts it moves downwards. The right crus of the diaphragm is attached to the upper three lumbar vertebrae. The diaphragm develops from a number of structures including the septum transversum, 4th cervical myotome, pleuroperitoneal membranes, thoracic wall and body wall dorsal to the suprarenal and mesonephric ridge.

**8  C E**
The pericardium consists of an outer fibrous and inner serous pericardium. The serous has two layers, and outer parietal lining and attached to the fibrous, and an inner visceral attached to the heart wall. It is also called the epicardium. The oblique sinus is behind the heart and is posterior to the left atrium. The transverse sinus is behind the aorta and pulmonary trunk and in front of the superior vena cava.

# Answers and Explanations Practice Exam 2

**9 A B D E**
Joints are usually supplied by nerves crossing them. The capitulum articulates with the head of the radius. The anastomosis round the elbow joint from which the joint receives its blood supply receives branches from the arteries named and also branches from the interosseous arteries.

**10 A C D**
The popliteal fossa is bounded above by the diverging hamstring muscles, laterally the biceps femoris and medially the semimembranosus and semitendinosus muscles; and below by the converging heads of the gastrocnemius muscle. Running downwards, more or less in the middle, are from superficial to deep the tibial nerve, the popliteal vein and the popliteal artery. Laterally, the common peroneal nerve is medial and often deep to the biceps femoris and is superficial to the lateral head of the gastrocnemius lower down.

**11 A B E**
The deep perineal space is between the perineal membrane (inferior fascia of the urogenital diaphragm) and the superior fascia of the urogenital diaphragm. The space contains the membranous urethra and sphincter urethrae muscle which formerly was called the external urethral sphincter. The internal urethral sphincter is now called the sphincter vesicae. The space also contains the bulbo-urethral glands whose ducts perforate the peroneal membrane and open into the spongy urethra. The superficial perineal pouch contains the bulb and crura of the penis and their related muscles, bulbospongiosus and ischiocavernosus.

**12 A B C**
The inferior rectal veins go to the pudendal vein in the pudendal canal on the lateral wall of the fossa. The canal contains the internal pudendal vessels and the pudendal nerve and is formed by a splitting of the fascia covering the obturator internus muscle on the lateral wall. The roof is formed by the sloping inferior surface of the levator ani muscle covered by fascia. The name 'ischiorectal' is a misnomer because the anal canal and its external sphincter form the medial wall. The fossa contains a considerable amount of lobulated fat.

## Answers and Explanations Practice Exam 2

**13 B E**

The common peroneal nerve divides into the superficial peroneal (musculocutaneous) nerve which supplies the peroneus longus and brevis muscles, and the deep peroneal (anterior tibial) nerve which supplies the extensor hallucis longus, extensor digitorum longus, peroneus tertius, tibialis anterior and extensor digitorum brevis muscles. The sides of all the toes are supplied by branches of either the deep or superficial peroneal nerves. The peroneal muscles are the only evertors of the foot. Tibialis posterior is an invertor and is not paralysed since it is supplied by the tibial nerve. All the dorsiflexors of the foot and toes are paralysed.

**14 B D E**

The parotid duct opens into the vestibule of the mouth inside the cheek opposite the upper 2nd molar tooth. The preganglionic secretomotor fibres leave the glossopharyngeal nerve in the jugular foramen and enter the petrous temporal. They leave as the lesser petrosal nerve. This nerve emerges from the bone inside the skull in the middle cranial fossa and leaves through or near the foramen ovale to end in the otic ganglion where it synapses with the postganglionic neurons. These postganglionic fibres join the auriculotemporal nerve and supply the parotid gland. The parotid gland is wedge-shaped with the sharp edge of the wedge going medially between the angle of the jaw and the mastoid process to reach the styloid process. At the angle of the jaw, part of the parotid gland lies medial to the mandible and becomes related to the medial pterygoid muscle.

**15 A B D E**

The pelvic diaphragm consists of the levator ani and coccygeus muscles on each side. It is attached to bone anteriorly (the posterior surface of the body of the pubis) and posteriorly (the ischial spine). Between these attachments it is attached to the obturator internus fascia. The fibres of the diaphragm pass medially and are attached to the coccyx and anococcygeal body, pass round the rectum, enter the perineal body (pass round the vagina) and become attached to the prostate (the bladder and beginning of the urethra in the female). Some of the fibres round the rectum continue downwards in the wall of the rectum and anal canal, mingle with the longitudinal muscle and split up the subcutaneous part of the external anal sphincter. The pelvic diaphragm contracts during coughing to prevent the contents of hollow organs passing downwards.

## Answers and Explanations Practice Exam 2

**16 A**
The spleen lies behind the stomach and in front of the left kidney. The right vagus nerve goes mainly to the posterior wall of the stomach and the left to the anterior wall. The vagus supplies the secretomotor fibres to the stomach. The oblique layer of muscle is internal to the other two. The splenic artery running along the upper border of the pancreas is a direct posterior relation of the stomach.

**17 A B C**
The ventral ramus of the 1st lumbar spinal nerve gives off the iliohypogastric and ilio-inguinal nerves and a branch to the genitofemoral nerve. The ilio-inguinal nerve is a mixed nerve and supplies the muscles of the lower abdominal wall and the skin in the pubic region and of the adjacent external genitalia-scrotum, labia majora and penis near the abdomen. The nerve runs deep to the external oblique muscle just above the inguinal ligament so that it enters the inguinal canal without passing through the deep ring.

**18 B C**
The pelvic splanchnic nerves are parasympathetic preganglionic nerves and are branches of the ventral (anterior primary) rami of the 2nd, 3rd and 4th sacral nerves. They supply preganglionic motor fibres to the smooth muscle of the pelvic viscera and the colon beyond the left colic (splenic) flexure. These fibres synapse near or in the wall of the viscera. The vagus nerves supply the rest of the gastro-intestinal tract in the abdomen. The pelvic splanchnic nerves are vasodilator to the erectile tissue of the penis (clitoris).

**19 A C E**
Since the arch of the aorta passes as much backwards as to the left, it is useful to think of many of the structures related to it as being to the right and posterior or to the left and anterior. The left vagus and phrenic nerves are anterior and to the left and the bifurcation of the trachea, the oesophagus and left recurrent laryngeal nerve are to the right and posterior. The recurrent laryngeal nerve is inferior before becoming posterior. The aortic arch reaches upwards only as far as the middle of the manubrium. The ductus arteriosus passes from the left pulmonary artery to the aortic arch and becomes the ligamentum arteriosum after birth. It is medial to the recurrent laryngeal nerve.

## Answers and Explanations Practice Exam 2

**20 A B**
The psoas major muscle is an important structure on the posterior abdominal wall. Anterior to it there are the colic and gonadal vessels and ureter (in that order) which are anterior to the genitofemoral nerve emerging from its anterior surface. The lumbar plexus is formed in the substance of the muscle which has the obturator nerve and lumbosacral trunk emerging medially and all the other branches except the genitofemoral emerging laterally. It is supplied by the ventral rami of the 2nd and 3rd lumbar spinal nerves as they pass through it. The external iliac vessels are medial to the psoas muscle although they become anterior near the inguinal ligament.

**21 A B E**
The Fick principle may be used to determine lung blood flow, and hence cardiac output, from the uptake of oxygen or from the carbon dioxide given off. The cardiac output may be increased up to 40 l/min in exercise, but heart rate increase need not necessarily lead to increased cardiac output as the stroke volume may fall. Cardiac output decreases progressively with age. There is increased peripheral vasodilatation on exposure to high temperatures, so that the cardiac output is unlikely to fall.

**22 A B C D**
The genotype of the mother could be A or AO. Thus the offspring or an AB father and an A mother could be A, B, or AB. Equally, a rhesus positive parent could be homozygous or heterozygous for this characteristic so that the children could be rhesus positive or rhesus negative.

**23 B C**
The oxygen dissociation curve is a plot of the percentage saturation of haemoglobin with oxygen against partial pressure of oxygen. A shift of the oxygen-haemoglobin dissociation curve to the left is produced by an increase in the affinity of oxygen as seen in cirrhosis of the liver. Anaemia, increased hydrogen ion concentration and an increase in $pCO_2$ are all associated with a decrease in oxygen affinity.

**24 A C**
Increasing the respiratory $CO_2$ to 5% causes a fall in the pH arterial blood and cerebrospinal fluid and hence respiratory stimulation. The oxygen-haemoglobin dissociation curve is shifted to the left so that the haemoglobin carries less oxygen at a given $pCO_2$ but the oxygen tension will be unaffected if the partial pressure of oxygen in the lungs does not alter. Cutaneous vasodilatation not vasoconstriction is seen.

## Answers and Explanations Practice Exam 2

**25 A B**
The airways resistance depends largely on the small peripheral airways because of their small diameter and large overall cross sectional area. Adrenaline and increased sympathetic activity dilate the bronchi, reducing resistance, while parasympathetic stimulation constricts the bronchi and increases resistance. The resistance depends on the lung volume and is greater on expiration, not inspiration.

**26 A B C D**
A relatively small amount of work is expanded in respiration at rest, being of the order of 4J (0.4kg.m) per min. About 60% is elastic work and 40% in overcoming viscous resistance. This is greater if the elastic recoil is greater or if there is narrowing of the bronchi. The compliance of the lungs is greater at volumes above the normal tidal range so that in this situation the work of respiration is increased. The surfactant diminishes the effect of surface tension in the alveoli, thus reducing the work of respiration.

**27 B C D E**
Plasma proteins serve a great variety of functions, but are not taken up by cells and used as metabolic fuel. Their functions do include control of plasma volume and carriage of various substances including carbon dioxide and hormones. Certain plasma proteins serve specific functions as for example immunity (immunoglobulins) and blood coagulation (fibrinogen).

**28 B D**
Large amounts of triglyceride are stored in the adipose tissue. This tissue is thus a source of relatively water-free fuel that is metabolically in a constant dynamic state.

**29 B C**
The increased secretion of mucous and enzymes occurring during the cephalic phase of digestion is mediated via the vagus. The excitatory effect of vagal stimulation occurs mainly by direct stimulation of the secretory cells, but also by indirect stimulation of the cells via gastrin. The sight and smell of food stimulate the release of gastric juices. The cephalic phase of digestion lasts longer than 5 minutes.

## Answers and Explanations Practice Exam 2

**30  A C D E**
Malabsorption of fats leading to their excretion in the faeces (steatorrhoea) may be due either to deficient secretion of bile salt or pancreatic lipase. The former can result either from hepatocellular failure or obstruction of flow from the gall bladder. Defective absorption of fats may also result from disease of the small intestinal mucosa as for example in coeliac disease. The stomach does not contribute significantly to the absorption of lipids.

**31  A B D**
Removal of large parts of the stomach will lead to achlorhydria. Anaemia also results because of the interference with intrinsic factor formation and hence vitamin $B_{12}$ absorption. After a meal in such patients there is a fall in plasma volume as fluid enters the gastrointestinal tract, contributing to the dumping syndrome. Blood glucose is elevated at the same time, but does not appear to contribute to the syndrome.

**32  A C D**
In order to measure renal plasma flow and hence renal blood flow, it is necessary to use a substance which is freely filtered and secreted, but not reabsorbed. Renal blood flow is 1/5 - 1/4 of the total cardiac output in normal conditions and is reduced in exercise when large amounts of blood flow through the muscles. Autoregulation occurs so that blood flow is constant over the blood pressure range 12-27 kPa (90-200 mmHg).

**33  A B E**
The excretion of drugs depends on their chemical nature, but the excretion is not usually greater because they are not ionized or are lipid soluble. Drugs such as PAH and penicillin are actively secreted into the urine in the proximal tubule. Excretion of such week anions may be inhibited by various substances. Probenic acid has been used to inhibit penicillin excretion. Excretion of drugs may cover the range of possible renal clearances.

**34  A D**
Ingestion of a large volume of water results in reduction of the plasma osmolality with a resultant fall in the activity of the neurohypophysial neurones and reduced vasopressin secretion. Excretion of the water load occurs over a period of a few hours. As the plasma osmolality falls, so water passes into the interstitial spaces. It is possible that the increase in blood volume will lead to stimulation of the atrial receptors, but not the chemoreceptors which are sensitive to changes in blood gas tensions.

## Answers and Explanations Practice Exam 2

**35 A B C E**
Both glucocorticoids and aldosterone are produced by the adrenal cortex, not the medulla. They are synthesized from cholesterol and are necessary for life.

**36 B C**
Parathyroid hormone is a single chain polypeptide containing 84 amino acids; it is the anterior pituitary which secretes a number of glycoprotein hormones. In physiological concentrations the main action of PTH is to increase calcium reabsorption in the renal tubule. With higher concentrations in the plasma there is reduced phosphate reabsorption by the renal tubule and increased calcium absorption in the intestine. This latter is not a direct action, but is mediated via 1.25-dihydroxycholecalciferol.

**37 A C D E**
The hypothalamus is the site of synthesis of posterior pituitary hormones and of hormones which control secretion from the anterior pituitary, being carried there via the portal blood system. It is also the site of receptors of blood temperature, but not of the pneumotaxic centre which lies in the pons. They hypothalamus shares a common embryological origin with the pituitary stalk and the posterior pituitary which also comprises nervous tissue.

**38 D**
Neurotransmitters are released from the presynaptic terminal when the action potentials arrive at the terminal. The two main neurotransmitters are catecholamines and acetylcholine, neither of which are peptides. Following synthesis in the presynaptic neurones they are stored in vesicles. When noradrenaline is released some combines with receptor sites postsynaptically and some is taken up again by the nerve terminals or is destroyed by enzymes located in the mitochondria or cytoplasm. After acetylcholine is released it is destroyed by acetylcholinesterase, ie. acetylcholinesterase found both in pre-and post-junctional cells.

**39 B C**
The knee jerk response is a stretch reflex and can be elicited by tapping the patella tendon, which stimulates the muscle spindle IA afferents. The reflex is monosynaptic, not involving any interneurones. Acetylcholine is involved as a transmitter. A pendular knee jerk is seen in a patient with an acute cerebellar lesion.

## Answers and Explanations Practice Exam 2

**40 D E**
The photosensitive cells, the rods and the cones lie in the outermost layer of the retina and are arranged side by side except for the central fovea where only cones are found. Overall the retina contains more rods than cones and possesses two blood supplies, a central retinal artery and a separate choroidal system of vessels. The image on the retina is inverted. Excessive illumination can produce damage.

**41 A B E**
Leukaemia is associated with some congenital disorders, particularly Down's syndrome, exposure to ionising radiation and cancer-chemotherapeutic drugs, and benzene poisoning. Phenylbutazone causes aplastic anaemia.

**42 C D**
The large bowel reabsorbs urinary hydrogen ions (causing a metabolic acidosis) and sodium chloride (causing hypernatraemia). Potassium is exchanged in the colon for sodium, leading to potassium depletion.

**43 A C**
Bone marrow supression is proportional to the dose of vincristine and mustine. Benzene and phenylbutazone have a high risk, and penicillin a low risk of idiosynchratic bone marrow suppression.

**44 D E**
The Kahn, W. R. and V. D. R. L. are all non-specific tests, also positive in a variety of other diseases (and in some healthy individuals). They demonstrate the presence of antibodies to 'cardiolipin' or similar lipid substances.

**45 A B C**
Polycythaemia may be due to reduced oxygenation of the blood, abnormal haemoglobin, tumours of kidney, uterine fibroids, cerebeller tumours and polycystic kidney disease.

**46 B D E**
Medullary carcinoma is a tumour of parafollicular or C cells of the thyroid, which produce calcitonin. It is familial in 5% of cases. It is associated with phaeochromocytoma, neuromas and parathyroid neoplasia in some patients. The tumour cells cause local amyloid deposition.

99

# Answers and Explanations Practice Exam 2

**47 C E**

*Streptococcus pyogenes* (group A α haemolytic Streptococci) causes throat infections, impetigo and erysipelas. If erythrogenic toxins are produced scarlet fever develops. Hypersensitivity reactions may also occur 2 - 3 weeks after infection, as an acute glomerulonephritis or rheumatic fever.

**48 A D E**

In hereditary cases it is transmitted as an autosomal dominant with variable penetrance. Retinoblastomas are derived from ectoderm, and commonly arise as bilateral primaries.

**49 A C D E**

Reactive thrombocythaemia occurs after trauma. Platelets are often raised at some stage in the chronic myeloproliferative disorders, but not in the acute leukaemias. The Schilling test involves saturation of $B_{12}$ stores by parenteral $B_{12}$ administration, and there may be a subsequent reactive overswing in circulating platelets in patients previously deficient in $B_{12}$

**50 A B C D**

Spirochaetes of medical importance belong to the genera Treponema (syphilis, yaws) Leptospira (Weil's disease, icterohaemorrhagic fever) and Borrelia (Vincent's organisms, found in large numbers in the lesions of Vincent's angina).

**51 C E**

Berry aneurysms are associated with a congenital defect in the media of arteries of the circle of Willis. Similar aneurysms on cerebral vessels are rarely due to syphilis and atherosclerosis. Aneurysms are found in both normotensive and hypertensive patients.

**52 A B C**

The male:female ratio is 10:1. The majority of laryngeal carcinomas arise on the vocal cords. Less than 5 per cent are adenocarcinomas, presumably of local mucus glands; the bulk are squamous carcinomas. Peak incidence is in the seventh decade.

**53 A B C D**

Down's syndrome is usually due to trisomy 21, although occasionally it is due to a translocation which effectively causes trisomy 21 with a normal chromosome number. There is an increased incidence of leukaemia. Webbing of the neck is a feature of Turner's syndrome.

*Answers and Explanations Practice Exam 2*

**54 B C**
Red infarcts occur in organs or tissue in which there is space for engorgement by blood from the venous side after arterial occlusion. Pale infarcts occur in tissues whose solid structure limits venous dilatation.

**55 B D E**
Amyloid is an eosinophilic material often derived from a circulating plasma protein or from immunoglobulin, or more rarely from other substances (eg. hormone fragments). Rectum is a useful biopsy site for diagnosis since the gastrointestinal tract is frequently involved.

**56 A B D**
Origin is from ovary (usually benign) or testis (usualy malignant), but can be from mediastinum, retroperitoneum, or intracranial (pineal). They represent tumours of a totipotent cell, and HCG production is associated with rapid metastasis and therapeutic resistance.

**57 A B C**
Sagittal sinus thrombosis causes hydrocephalus through interference with CSF reabsorption via the arachnoid granulations. Gardiner's syndrome is an autosomal dominant condition consisting of polyposis coli, together with multiple epidermoid cysts and osteomas.

**58 A C E**
*Yersinia pestis*, the agent of plague, is a flea-borne pathogen of rodents. So far as is known, man is the only reservoir for *Vibrio cholerae*. The reservoir of yellow fever is the monkey. Epidemic typhus has a human reservoir, a louse vector. Endemic typhus is primarily a disease of rats. Leishmaniasis has both human and non-human reservoirs.

**59 A B**
Aspartate transaminase is present in high activity in cardiac and skeletal muscle, liver and kidney.

**60 C D E**
Pick's disease follows tuberculous pericarditis, which leads to congestive heart failure. In Meigs's syndrome an ovarian fibroma is associated with ascites. In pseudomyxoma peritonei the peritoneal cavity becomes filled with mucus.

# ANSWERS TO PRACTICE EXAM 3

**1  A E**

Damage to the upper trunk (C5, 6) produces a paralysis of the muscles supplied by these roots. The movements lost at the shoulder joint are abduction and lateral rotation. Flexion at the shoulder joint is almost completely lost. Flexion and supination of the forearm are lost. Muscles paralysed include the deltoid, supraspinatus, infraspinatus, teres minor, biceps brachii, brachialis, supinator and brachioradialis.

**2  A D E**

The glossopharyngeal nerve emerges from the skull through the jugular foramen which lies between the occipital and petrous temporal bones. It contains fibres of general sensation from the posterior part of the tongue and most of the lining of the pharynx, taste fibres from the posterior part of the tongue and also the vallate papillae, and sensory fibres from the carotid sinus and body. The nerve also contains motor fibres to the stylopharyngeus muscle and preganglionic parasympathetic fibres which synapse in the otic ganglion. The postganglionic fibres go to the parotid gland.

**3  A**

The internal spermatic fascia is derived from the transversalis fascia. The transversus abdominis muscle may contribute a few fibres to the cremasteric fascia derived mainly from the internal oblique muscle. The lymphatic vessels in the spermatic cord come from the testis and epididymis and go to the iliac and para-aortic nodes. The vessels from the scrotum go to the superficial inguinal nodes. The superficial inguinal ring has a base medial to the pubic tubercle and two sides (crura) which pass upwards and laterally so that the spermatic cord as it passes into the scrotum at the base of the ring is medial to the tubercle.

**4  A B C E**

The sciatic nerve is in two parts before it divides into the tibial (medial popliteal) and common peroneal (lateral popliteal) nerves. The tibial part supplies the long head of biceps femoris, semimembranosus and semitendinosus, and the common peroneal part supplies the short head of the biceps. The tibial nerve divides into the lateral and medial plantar nerves. The medial plantar nerve supplies the abductor hallucis muscle. The tibial nerve gives articular branches to the knee joint.

## Answers and Explanations Practice Exam 3

**5 B C D E**
The biceps femoris muscle has a long head which is attached with the semitendinosus to the ischial tuberosity medial to the attachment of the semimembranosus. The short head is attached to the linea aspera of the femur. The common peroneal nerve is medial and usually deep to the biceps femoris in the popliteal fossa and winds round the neck of the fibula 1-2 cm distal to the attachment. The biceps femoris can rotate the leg at the knee joint if the knee is partly flexed. In the fully extended knee this movement is impossible.

**6 A B C E**
The neural tube is closed by the end of the 4th week. Herniation of part of the midgut is present at about the 5th week and normally is absent by the end of the 12th week. The limb buds are seen by the 4th week. The palatine processes appear in the 6th week and fuse in the 7th week. The mandibular processes appear in the 4th week and fuse by the 5th week.

**7 B E**
The deltoid muscle is innervated by the axillary nerve which contains fibres from the 5th and 6th cervical spinal nerves. Its middle part (from the acromion) is multipennate and its anterior (from the clavicle) and posterior (from the scapular spine) parts are unipennate. The middle part is an abductor at the shoulder joint but for initiation requires an intact supraspinatus muscle. The anterior fibres flex and medially rotate at the shoulder joint and the posterior fibres extend and laterally rotate.

**8 B C E**
The anterior lobe (adenohypophysis) is derived from the roof of the stomatodeum (Rathke's pouch) and is ectodermal. The posterior lobe (neurohypophysis) is derived from the neural tube which is also ectodermal in origin. The superior and inferior hypophyseal arteries come from the internal carotid and there is a complicated system of portal veins in the gland linking the capillaries of the median eminence and infundibulum with the capillaries of the neuro- and adenohypophysis. The gland is inferior to the optic chiasma.

**9 B D E**
The right border is formed by the right atrium and the left border by the left ventricle. The right ventricle forms most of the anterior surface of the heart. The pulmonary artery at its origin is anterior and to the left of the ascending aorta. Only the left auricle (auricular appendage) of the left atrium can be seen from the front, to the left of the pulmonary artery.

# Answers and Explanations Practice Exam 3

**10 A B C**

The radial nerve is the largest branch of the brachial plexus and is a continuation of the posterior cord. The nerve lies on the muscles forming the posterior wall of the axilla behind the axillary artery and then behind the humerus in the groove for the radial nerve. It appears anteriorly in a groove between the brachioradialis and brachialis muscles in the region of the elbow. The radial nerve gives off the posterior cutaneous nerves of the upper arm and forearm as well as the lower lateral cutaneous nerve of the upper arm. At the elbow it divides into a superficial and deep branch (the former was known as the radial nerve in the forearm and the latter as the posterior interosseous nerve). The superficial branch is sensory to the skin of the back of the lateral three and a half digits as far as the distal interphalangeal joint.

**11 A B D E**

The preganglionic sympathetic fibres come from the 1st thoracic segment of the spinal cord and travel in the 1st intercostal nerve, then in its white ramus communicans and upwards in the cervical part of the sympathetic ganglionated trunk to the superior cervical ganglion where they synapse. The postganglionic sympathetic fibres have their cell bodies in that ganglion and enter the skull with the internal carotid artery. They reach the orbit and eyeball via the cavernous sinus and superior orbital fissure and supply blood vessels and the dilator pupillae. The preganglionic parasympathetic fibres are in the oculomotor nerve and go to the ciliary ganglion. The postganglionic parasympathetic fibres have their cell bodies in that ganglion and innervate the ciliary muscle and sphincter pupillae.

**12 B C D E**

The skin of the pinna and external acoustic meatus is innervated by the auriculotemporal (a branch of the mandibular), great auricular and vagus nerves. The tympanic membrane on its outer surface is innervated by the auriculotemporal and vagus nerves and by the glossopharyngeal nerve on its inner surface. The external acoustic meatus is straightened by pulling the pinna upwards and backwards because the meatus curves upwards and backwards as it passes medially. With the aural speculum and good light the tympanic membrane, the handle of the malleus and long process of the incus can usually be seen.

## Answers and Explanations Practice Exam 3

**13 B C E**
The superficial perineal pouch contains the bulb of the penis (vestibular bulbs) and the crura of the penis (crura of the clitoris) and their respective muscles, the bulbospongiosus and ischiocavernosus. The greater vestibular glands (female) and bulbourethral glands (male) are homologous but the greater vestibular glands are in the superficial pouch and the bulbo-urethral glands in the deep pouch. The duct of the bulbo-urethral gland pierces the perineal membrane and opens into the urethra in the corpus spongiosum. There are transverse perineal muscles in both the superficial and deep pouches, and the (external) sphincter of the urethra is in the deep pouch.

**14 A B E**
The arteries running along the lesser curvature are the left gastric from the coeliac and the right gastric from the hepatic. The arteries along the greater curvature are the left gastro-epiploic from the splenic and the right gastro-epiploic from the gastroduodenal, a branch of the hepatic. The omental bursa is posterior to the stomach and the spleen is wedged between the stomach anteriorly and the left kidney posteriorly. The left vagus nerve goes mainly to the anterior surface and the right to the posterior surface.

**15 A C**
There is a vertical ridge on the posterior wall of the prostatic urethra on which the prostatic utricle opens. The utricle extends upwards deep to the crest. The median lobe is defined as that part of the prostate posterior to the urethra and between the common ejaculatory ducts. The stroma of the prostate is fibromuscular. Its venous plexus is outside its own capsule and deep to its pelvic fascial covering. The peripheral glands of the prostate are large and branched and are associated with carcinoma of the gland. The glands near the urethra are shorter and are involved in benign hypertrophy.

**16 A B C E**
Each extensor expansion has a lumbrical muscle attached to its lateral side distal to the interosseous muscle. The expansion has on each side an interosseous muscle. That of the index finger has the 1st dorsal interosseous (lateral) and the 2nd palmar (medial); the ring finger has the 3rd palmer (lateral) and the 4th dorsal (medial) interosseous. The little finger has the 4th palmar (lateral) and the abductor digiti minimi (medial). There is no synovial sheath for the extensor expansion.

# Answers and Explanations Practice Exam 3

**17 A C E**
The position of the aortic sinuses is different in the fetus (two anterior and one posterior) from that in the adult (one anterior and two posterior). The adult arrangement should be used. The right coronary artery lies betwen the right atrium and pulmonary trunk. The blood supply of the sino-atrial node can be derived from either the right coronary (60%) or left coronary (40%) artery. Some branches of the right coronary artery supply the left atrium and left ventricle adjacent to the corresponding right chambers. The left coronary artery, supplying much more myocardium than the right, is usually of a larger calibre.

**18 B C D**
The midgut extend from the middle of the duodenum (descending or 2nd part just distal to the common opening of the bile and pancreatic ducts) to the transverse colon proximal to the left colic flexure. Its artery is the superior mesenteric which acts as the axis of rotation of the midgut. The rotation is in a counterclockwise direction. The embryonic herniation consists mainly of midgut.

**19 A B D**
There are usually 7 permanent teeth in each quadrant by 14 years. The 3rd molar may erupt between about 17 and 25 years. The first permanent tooth to erupt is usually the 1st permanent molar at about 6 years (6th year molar) but in many children the lower central incisor may be the first to erupt.

**20 D**
Postganglionic sympathetic fibres are found in peripheral nerves and in the plexuses round blood vessels. The short ciliary nerves contain sensory or postganglionic sympathetic or parasympathetic fibres. Preganglionic sympathetic fibres from the 1st thoracic to the 1st lumbar spinal cord segments enter the sympathetic ganglionated trunk and some of them leave the trunk in the splanchnic nerves without synapsing. Preganglionic fibres are small myelinated (white) and postganglionic are non-myelinated (grey).

**21 B D**
The aortic and pulmonary valves each have three semilunar cusps of very thin fibrous tissue covered by endocardium. The chordae tendinae are connected to the a-v valves, not the aortic valve. The three pockets of the valve meet down three lines and prevent blood flow back into the ventricle. With inadequate closure or incompetence the blood regurgitates back leading to a high pulse pressure, not a low systolic pressure.

## Answers and Explanations Practice Exam 3

**22 B C D**
A decrease in the affinity of haemoglobin for oxygen is seen in pregnancy, in residents at high altitude, with a rise in temperature and a fall in pH (rise in H+). In the presence of diphosphoglycerate (DPG) the reduced form of haemoglobin is stabilised and the affinity of haemoglobin for oxygen is greatly diminished.

**23 B C E**
The flow rate of blood in the aorta is greater than in the capillaries which have a greater cross sectional area. Carbon dioxide is added to the blood in the capillaries so that the pH falls. The carbon dioxide diffuses into the red blood cells where, under the influence of carbonic anhydrase, bicarbonate is formed, which subsequently moves out of the red cells. Chloride ions move in to maintain electrical neutrality.

**24 B C E**
The P wave coincides with the depolarisation of the atria and the R wave with depolarisation of the apex of the heart - representing the plateau region of the action potential in the ventricles. The upper limit of normal for the P-R interval is 0.2 secs. Ventricular systole is of much longer duration than the QRS complex, lasting until repolarisation which occurs at the T wave.

**25 A E**
Type II alveolar cells produce a phospholipoprotein complex known as pulmonary surfactant. It prevents smaller alveoli collapsing into larger ones, so alteration of surface tension to the same degree would not be effective. It is formed in fetal life and sometimes, especially in premature births, if insufficient is available or if it is inactive then the neonatal respiratory distress syndrome is seen.

**26 A**
The functional residual capacity (FRC) is nearly 3.0l and is measured using a helium dilution technique. As the resistance to flow increases so a new equilibrium is established with the lung pulled to a higher volume so the FRC tends to decrease. In the healthy individual the airways begin to close as the residual volume is approached.

## Answers and Explanations Practice Exam 3

**27 A B C**
Blood or plasma volume may be determined using dilution techniques. Suitable substances for use in this approach include harmless dyes such as rose bengal and Evans blue. Albumin labelled with radioactive iodine has also been used and labelled red cells. Deuterium oxide is used to determine total body water and inulin to determine extracellular fluid volume and glomerular filtration rate.

**28 C D**
During exercise blood glucose is initially maintained or even increased as a result of a greater production rate involving inter alia gluconeogenesis stimulated by circulating catecholamines. The anaerobic component of metabolism leads to the release of lactate resulting in increased plasma lactate and a fall in plasma pH. Muscle glycogen stores are depleted in exercise, but only if the work is very severe. Increased ventilation during exercise helps to keep the $PaCO_2$ normal initially. It decreases if the anaerobic threshold is reached.

**29 A B C D**
In some people the gliadin in wheat produces damage of the intestinal mucosa so that the villi disappear especially in the upper small intestine. The condition manifests itself as coeliac disease in children and steatorrhoea in adults. The impaired absorption in the small intestine results in reduced bile acid secretion, steatorrhoea and macrocytic anaemia, as well as many other features of a malabsorption syndrome. The condition may be treated by a gluten-free diet.

**30 B C D**
Secretin is a polypeptide comprising 17 amino acids, its major action being stimulation of water and electrolytes from the pancreas. It is only a weak stimulant of enzyme secretion. It exerts a negative feedback in man to reduce gastric secretion motility and emptying. It also stimulates biliary secretion.

**31 A B E**
Segmentation occurs throughout the length of the small intestine and is highly efficient in mixing chyme with digestive juices. Also, because there is a graded frequency with a higher rate in the upper part of the intestine, the chyme is moved from the upper part to the lower part.

## Answers and Explanations Practice Exam 3

**32 A C E**
Glucose is filtered at the glomerulus and actively reabsorbed by the proximal tubule by a process involving co-transport with sodium and which is blocked by phlorizin. Glucose appears in the urine during diabetes mellitus and can cause an increase in urine flow.

**33 A B C D**
Receptors exist within the cardiovascular tree which respond to changes in volume and arterial pressure and which, by various routes can influence secretion of hormones important in regulating the extra-cellular fluid volume, vasopressin by promoting water reabsorption and aldosterone by promoting sodium reabsorption. Factor IV is the name sometimes applied to calcium in regard to blood clotting mechanisms. The factor postulated to be involved in sodium excretion (but not definitely proven) is the third factor or natriuretic factor.

**34 B C**
The normal healthy adult produces about 1.5l urine daily, containing 50g solids, the chief constituents being urea and sodium chloride. Comparatively less creatinine is excreted and under normal conditions glucose is totally reabsorbed by the kidney.

**35 B C D**
Insulin is synthesised in the $\beta$ cells of the pancreatic islands (islets of Langerhans). It acts to reduce blood glucose concentrations, stimulating uptake into muscle and facilitating glycogen synthesis in liver and muscle. It also produces an increase in protein synthesis and inhibits release of non-esterified fatty acids from fat depots.

**36 B E**
Steroid hormones do not bind to receptors in the cell membrane, neither do they produce increased intracellular concentrations of cyclic AMP. They act mainly by entering the cell, binding to receptor proteins within the cytosol. The hormone receptor complex then enters the nucleus where it influences the synthesis of specific proteins.

**37 B**
It is believed that contraceptive pills containing oestrogen and progesterone suppress the release of the gonadotrophins, luteinising hormone (LH) and follicular stimulating hormone (FSH) and thus prevent ovulation. They also alter the composition of the cervical mucous so that spermatozoa may fail to penetrate the uterine cavity.

## Answers and Explanations Practice Exam 3

**38 A B C**
Vasopressin is synthesised in the magnocellular nuclei (supraoptic and paraventricular nuclei) in the hypothalamus. It is released from the posterior pituitary in response to a number of stimuli including volume depletion, as in haemorrhage. Release is pulsatile and a diurnal rhythm is also seen. It has a short half time in plasma of less than 10 minutes. It acts on the collecting duct to produce an increase in cyclic AMP and a consequent increase in tubular permeability and increased water retention.

**39 A B C D**
The thick filaments are comprised entirely of myosin. Troponin and actin are found in the thin filaments. In the process of stimulus excitation coupling calcium ions are released from the lateral sacs of the sarcoplasmic reticulum and these ions subsequently bind to troponin located on the thin filaments so that the active sites on the actin are uncovered and cross bridges formed. To break the cross bridge a small amount of ATP is split to ADP. The energy from ATP is not used directly in force production, but is used to alter the state of the cross bridge.

**40 A E**
Shivering never occurs below the lesion in spinal man. Abdominal reflexes are also lost as they depend on the integrity of the corticospinal projection. Micturition is a spinal reflex and is still present, but the person will have an automatic bladder. Tendon jerks are potentiated in the affected area. Sweating is not lost, but can be markedly augmented as a result of uncontrolled sympathetic activity.

**41 C E**
IgM consists of 5 four-chain units, the units consisting of light and heavy chains. The heavy chain is of a type specific for IgM. IgM does not cross the placenta. It is the earliest class of Ig produced. Rheumatoid factor consists largely of IgM anti-IgG antibody. IgG is the commonest antibody class in serum.

**42 A C D**
Folic acid and vitamin $B_{12}$ deficiency (pernicious anaemia) are associated with normochromic macrocytic red cells. Chronic inflammatory diseases, thalassaemia and iron deficiency are all associated with hypochromic microcytic red cells.

## Answers and Explanations Practice Exam 3

**43 A B D E**
Increased plasma cholesterol is often seen in myxoedema, biliary obstruction, nephrotic syndrome, diabetes and chronic renal failure.

**44 C D E**
*Streptococcus pyogenes* is a synonym for group A streptococci, which are $\beta$ haemolytic. The organism forms chains in culture, and may form an erythrogenic toxin which causes scarlet fever. Sometimes erythema nodosum develops after infection by *S. pyogenes*.

**45 C D**
Patients who have had chickenpox harbour quiescent virus in nerve bodies, which may be reactivated, especially in immunosuppressed patients, as herpes zoster. Virus will then be present in vesicles and they may cause chicken pox in contacts.

**46 B C D**
Adenolymphomas are virtually restricted to elderly men; almost all arise in the parotid gland; they are benign, and consist of a mixture of eosinophilic epithelium and lymphoid tissue.

**47 B C E**
In pyloric stenosis there is loss of gastric hydrogen ions, chloride ions and water. This causes haemoconcentration and metabolic alkalosis. Potassium deficiency is caused by renal compensation.

**48 A D**
The spleen is usually very large in CLL, and patients commonly present with a sensation of left hypochondrial fullness, or pain from splenic infarcts. It is more common in males than females (2:1). The lymphocytes are usually $\beta$ cells, but they are not usually actively producing immunoglobulins.

**49 B C**
Diverticular disease characteristically affects the sigmoid colon, and only rarely involves the ascending and transverse colon. The disease is rare below 50. It is associated with muscle hypertrophy and mucosal outpouchings between muscle bands (false diverticula). The sex incidence is approximately equal.

**50 C D E**
Anaphylaxis and serum sickness are mediated by antibodies, formed by B cells. T cells are affector cells in delayed hypersensitivity and graft rejection, and are responsible for conversion from Mantoux negativity to Mantoux positivity.

## Answers and Explanations Practice Exam 3

**51 A C**
Nephroblastoma and medulloblastoma are tumours of childhood; teratomas of young adults.

**52 A B**
Crohn's disease may involve any part of the alimentary tract from lips to anus. It is characterised by transmural inflammation and fissuring ulceration, and because the transmural inflammation causes adhesions, it penetrates rather than perforates, to cause sinuses and fistulae instead. Granulomas are localised to the alimentary tract and draining lymph nodes.

**53 D**
Crohn's disease probably has a statistical association with carcinoma, but is such a rare complication as to be clinically not significant. Although diverticulosis and carcinoma of colon occur in similar populations, diverticulosis is so common that the finding of diverticular disease does not raise the suspicion of malignancy.

**54 A C**
The tumour typically spreads via the blood stream to produce osteosclerotic deposits. The lumbar vertebrae are particularly affected, possibly by a local portal system. The tumour tends to arise in different areas of the prostate from those in which adenomatous growths arise. Gynaecomastia may arise as a result of oestrogen therapy for the tumour.

**55 A**
The nephrotic syndrome is characteristically associated with the minimal change lesion, renal amyloid, membranous glomerulonephritis and diabetic glomerulosclerosis.

**56 A B C**
Even relatively minor unaccustomed exercise can cause an increase in serum creatine kinase levels. They are raised in patients with overt Duchenne's muscular dystrophy and also in carriers of the disease.

**57 B**
Phenylketonuria is inherited as an autosomal recessive character. It occurs once in about every 30,000 live births. The disease can be ameliorated if phenylalanine is removed from the diet very early in life.

## Answers and Explanations Practice Exam 3

**58  E**
Silica causes pulmonary fibrosis and right ventricular hypertrophy. Silicosis does not predispose to mesothelioma or bronchial carcinoma.

**59  A D E**
*Clostridium tetani* is a strict anaerobe which can nevertheless grow in inconspicuous wounds. It remains localised and produces a neurotoxin which spreads along nerves. Symptoms commence days or even months after infection.

**60  D**
Unlike chronic granulocytic leukaemia, there is no terminal blastic phase in chronic lymphatic leukaemia. It is very rare below 35 years, and reaches a peak incidence in the 6th decade. Chronic myeloid leukaemia is usually associated with deletion of the long arm of chromosome 22 (ph chromosome). The disease has an equal sex ratio. Bilateral, painless swelling of salivary and lacrymal glands (Mikulicz's syndrome) is rare but a well-recognised feature.

# ANSWERS TO PRACTICE EXAM 4

1 **A B C E**
   The swallowing reflex is set up when the food stimulates the oropharynx whose mucous membrane is supplied by the glossopharyngeal nerve. The stylopharyngeus and palatopharyngeus muscles are attached to the thyroid cartilage and when they contract the larynx is raised. As the laryngeal opening approaches the epiglottis the aryepiglottis muscles contract and close the opening. The vocal folds are adducted. All the muscles of the pharynx, larynx and soft palate, except the tensor veli palatini are supplied by fibres whose cell bodies are in the nucleus ambiguus. The fibres are mainly in the cranial accessory nerve; some are in the vagus and glossopharyngeal nerves.

2 **B C D E**
   The posterior spinocerebellar tract enters in the inferior peduncle and the anterior in the superior peduncle. The inferior peduncle also contains vestibulocerebellar, olivocerebellar and cuneocerebellar fibres. The superior peduncle contains mainly fibres from the dentate nucleus to the red nucleus and thalamus. The oldest part of the cerebellum receives the vestibulocerebellar fibres. The palaeocerebellum, the newest part, receives the fibres from the pontine nuclei. These are acted on by the fronto- and temporopontine fibres from the cerebral cortex. The neocerebellum, regarded as intermediate between the other two, receives the spinocerebellar tracts.

3 **A D E**
   The posterior layer of the rectus sheath is present distal to the costal margin and ends as the arcuate line, approximately midway between the umbilicus and symphysis pubis. The lower intercostal nerves (6th - 11th) run horizontally in relation to the muscle. The tendinous intersections are attached to the anterior layer of the sheath and not to the posterior layer. The inguinal triangle, the lateral part of which is the site of a direct inguinal hernia, is bounded laterally by the inferior epigastric vessels and inferiorly by the inguinal ligament. The inferior epigastric artery from the external iliac anastomoses with the superior epigastric, a branch of the internal thoracic (mammary), a branch of the subclavian.

# Answers and Explanations Practice Exam 4

**4 A C D**

The lesser omentum is a double fold of peritoneum extending superiorly from the porta hepatis and fissure for the ligamentum venosum of the liver downwards to the lesser curvature of the stomach and the superior (1st) part of the duodenum. Its lateral free edge forms the anterior boundary of the epiploic foramen (aditus to the lesser sac) in which are the portal vein posteriorly and the (common) bile duct (right) and hepatic artery (left) anteriorly. The two layers separate at the lesser curvature of the stomach along which the gastric vessels run.

**5 A B E**

The obturator internus muscle is attached to the lateral wall of the pelvis. Its upper part is above the levator ani muscle and has the obturator nerve on its medial surface. Its lower part below the levator ani forms the lateral wall of the ischiorectal fossa and has the pudendal nerve on its medial surface. The tendon of the muscle leaves the pelvis through the lesser sciatic foramen and goes to the greater trochanter. The nerve to the muscle is from L5, S1, 2 mainly the 5th lumbar nerve.

**6 B C**

The macula is on the lateral side of the optic disc. Unlike the vitreous body, which is irreplaceable, the aqueous is continually secreted and absorbed. When focusing on near objects, the ciliary muscle contracts so that the suspensory ligament is relaxed and allows the lens to become more biconvex (accommodation). In detachment of the retina the separation takes place between the pigment layer and the rest of the retina. This is due to the way in which the retina develops from the optic vesicle and cup. There are only cones at the macula, the site of sharpest vision.

**7 A B**

The left phrenic nerve supplies the left half of the diaphragm but the right crus crosses to the left of the midline. The superior intercostal vein passes between the vagus and phrenic nerves. The vagus nerve is posterior and this is the relation of the nerves as they pass to the left of the arch of the aorta. The thoracic duct passes forwards at its termination. The phrenic nerve on both sides is anterior to the hilum. The transverse (superficial) cervical and suprascapular arteries "tie down" the phrenic nerve on to the scalenus anterior muscle as they pass laterally and backwards across that muscle.

## Answers and Explanations Practice Exam 4

**8 A B E**

The inferior epigastric artery arises from the external iliac artery just proximal to the inguinal ligament. It passes upwards and medially on the deep aspect of the anterior abdominal wall and forms the lateral boundary of the inguinal triangle which is crossed by the obliterated umbilical artery. It is therefore medial to the inferior epigastric artery. The inferior epigastric artery gives off pubic branches which may enlarge and form an abnormal obturator artery. The inferior epigastric artery lies between the posterior layer of the rectus sheath and the rectus abdominis muscle.

**9 C E**

The scalenus anterior is attached to the scalene tubercle and the suprapleural membrane is attached to the medial border of the 1st rib. Only the lower trunk of the brachial plexus is directly related to its upper surface behind the subclavian artery.

**10 B C D**

There are about 15-20 lobes, each of which has a separate lactiferous duct opening on to the nipple. The suspensory ligaments divide the breast into lobes and are extensions into the breast of the superficial fascia around the organ. The nipple has no sweat glands or hair follicles unlike the areola which has both. The enlargement of the breast at puberty is due to an increase in connective tissue and fat. The ducts elongate at puberty but glandular tissue develops in large amounts only during pregnancy.

**11 A B C E**

The peritoneum of the recto-uterine pouch (of Douglas) is related to the upper third of the posterior vaginal wall. The ureter passes forwards below the uterine artery lateral to the vagina near the cervix of the uterus. Anteriorly the peritoneum passes from the bladder to the uterus (vesico-uterine pouch) above the level of the vagina.

**12 B C D**

The median nerve is lateral to the axillary artery and its continuation the brachial artery. The nerve crosses anterior to the brachial artery about the middle of the upper arm and becomes medial to it at the elbow. The median nerve is adherent to the deep surface of the flexor digitorum superficialis and becomes more superficial just proximal to the wrist where the nerve lies between the palmaris longus and flexor carpi radialis tendons. The nerve is deep to the flexor retinaculum and its digital branches are deep to the superficial palmar arch.

# Answers and Explanations Practice Exam 4

**13  A**

The obturator nerve passes downwards and forwards on the lateral wall of the pelvis 1 cm below the brim to the upper part of the obturator membrane where the nerve passes into the thigh between the membrane and the bone. On the lateral wall of the pelvis the nerve passes lateral to the internal iliac artery and is the most external (lateral) of all the structures (ureter, gonadal vessels, round ligament or ductus deferens, obliterated umbilical artery). The obturator internus muscle has its own nerve supply from the sacral plexus (L5, S1, 2). The anterior branch has a cutaneous element which goes to the lower part of the medial side of the thigh.

**14  B D**

The hypoglossal nerve leaves the skull through the hypoglossal canal (anterior condyloid foramen). The internal vertebral venous plexus in the vertebral canal extends from the pelvis to within the cranium and with the external vertebral venous plexus (outside the bony vertebrae) provides a venous communication between all levels of the trunk and the intracranial sinuses. The spinal accessory nerve on each side from the upper cervical segments enters the skull through the foramen magnum and joins the cranial accessory. The accessory nerve leaves the skull through the jugular foramen. The outer layer of dura mater ends at the foramen magnum. The inner layer is continuous with the spinal dura through the foramen magnum.

**15  B C D**

The sciatic nerve is deep to the lower half of the gluteus maximus. It is lateral to the posterior femoral cutaneous nerve.

**16  A B D**

The serratus anterior is the most important muscle in pulling the scapula forwards and rotating it so that the glenoid cavity faces upwards. In the latter movement it is assisted by the upper fibres of the trapezius. The rhomboid muscles rotate the scapula so that the glenoid cavity faces downwards. The pectoralis minor assists in this movement because its line of pull on the coracoid process is inferior to the axis of rotation.

117

## Answers and Explanations Practice Exam 4

**17 B C E**
The pectineus muscle is medial to the psoas tendon which is medial to the iliacus muscle. In the femoral sheath, the femoral artery is lateral to the femoral vein which is lateral to the femoral canal. The femoral nerve is outside and lateral to the sheath. The femoral branch of the genitofemoral nerve is lateral to the femoral artery and pierces the sheath and fascia lata near the saphenous opening. The small superficial veins join the great (long) saphenous vein before it passes through the saphenous opening and joins the femoral vein.

**18 None correct**
As the ureter passes downwards on the psoas muscle it is anterior to the genitofemoral nerve and posterior to the gonadal vessels which are posterior to the colic vessels (right colic, left colic and ileocolic). The obturator nerve is the most external (lateral) of the structures on the pelvic wall. The ureter crosses the brim of the pelvis at the sacro-iliac joint from which it is separated by the division of the common iliac artery.

**19 B D E**
The femoral nerve ends as the saphenous nerve which runs in the adductor (subsartorial, Hunter's) canal, pierces its roof and continues down the medial side of the leg and foot. The lateral femoral cutaneous nerve is an independent branch of the lumbar plexus.

**20 A B C D**
The first aortic arch arteries disappear as do the second except for the dorsal part which forms part of the stapedial artery. The third arch artery forms the proximal part of the internal carotid. The right fourth aortic arch artery forms the proximal part of the subclavian artery and the left fourth forms part of the aortic arch. The fifth disappears. The sixth arch artery on the right disappears almost entirely but its ventral part forms part of the right pulmonary artery. The left sixth artery forms part of the pulmonary trunk and the ductus arteriosus.

**21 C D E**
Blood pressure has been given as
   blood pressure = cardiac output × peripheral resistance.
Therefore, it rises when peripheral resistance increases on exposure to cold. It falls when venous return falls as on assumption of the upright posture. It does not necessarily increase when heart rate increases as an increase in heart rate does not always produce an increase in cardiac output. Hypoxia acts on the pressor area in the medulla to give an increase in blood pressure. It also increases with age.

## Answers and Explanations Practice Exam 4

**22 A B D E**
Tissue fluid is formed as a result of the balance between hydrostatic pressure forcing fluid into the tissue and the osmotic pressure of the plasma which tends to draw fluid into the vascular space. Thus increased capillary pressure, as seen with arteriolar dilatation which may occur in hot weather or with increased pressure in the veins as in pregnancy, tends to force fluid out into the tissue. Likewise reduced plasma protein concentration results in reduced fluid returning to the vascular space. Filtration of fluid from the capillaries is generally greater than the gain of fluid, the excess being removed by the lymphatic system, so reduction of the efficiency of this system leads to oedema.

**23 A C E**
Hypercoagulability may contribute to intravascular clotting. However, it appears that the state of the blood vessel lining is more important. Such vessel oriented explanations can explain the increased probability of vascular thrombosis with stasis, inflammation or damage etc. of blood vessels and accumulation of lipids and smooth muscle cells in arterial walls. Blood coagulation requires calcium and fibrinogen and involves clumping of platelets.

**24 B C D**
The posterior pituitary nonapeptide vasopressin and the octapeptide angiotensin II are both powerful vasoconstrictors. Histamine, 5HT (serotonin) and bradykinin are all vasodilator substances.

**25 A C**
With voluntary over ventilation carbon dioxide is blown off so that the alveolar $pCO_2$ is reduced from the normal value of 5.3kPa (40mmHg). Arterial $pCO_2$ also falls so that the blood hydrogen ion concentration falls in accordance with the Henderson-Hasselbach equation
$$pH = 6.1 + \log_{10}|HCO_3-|/|CO_2 \text{ in solution}|$$
and the bicarbonate concentration increases to maintain the blood pH constant. The increased plasma pH results in a fall in plasma calcium and hence there is increased muscle excitability. The fall in $PaCO_2$ constricts the cerebral blood vessels so that the cerebral blood flow is reduced.

# Answers and Explanations Practice Exam 4

**26 A B C D E**
When the oxygen saturation of the blood falls as with impaired circulation or pulmonary oedema the $pO_2$ of the peripheral chemoreceptors falls and breathing is stimulated. When the oxygen saturation rises breathing diminishes or ceases. Cheyne-Stokes respiration also occurs in healthy people at high altitudes and after hyperventilation when $CO_2$ is blown off and respiration depressed.

**27 B D**
The liver receives the greater part of its blood supply from the hepatic portal system not from the hepatic artery. Thus on absorption amino acids and glucose pass to the liver where they are metabolised, glycogen and urea being amongst the products formed. The plasma proteins albumin and fibrinogen are primarily synthesised in the liver, but not immunoglobulins.

**28 B C E**
Pancreatic cells with endocrine function are found in small clumps (islets of Langerhans). Pancreatic exocrine cells form the greater mass of the cells. Exocrine secretions contain enzymes and much bicarbonate. Acetylcholine acts mainly on the acinar cells to cause release of enzymes, while secretin acts principally on centroacinar and duct cells to cause release of water and electrolytes.

**29 D E**
The jejunum is the main site of absorption of the products of digestion. Iron and fat soluble vitamins are also absorbed in this region, $B_{12}$ is absorbed in the ileum which is also the primary site of absorption of bile salts.

**30 B D E**
Following vagotomy the sensation of hunger is reduced, but not absent. The vagus nerve stimulates gastric acid secretion so vagotomy results in a fall in gastric acid secretion. It does not cause atrophy of the gastric mucosa. Vagotomy also prolongs emptying of the gall bladder and its resting size doubles. Reduced intestinal motility is seen.

**31 C D**
It was believed that urea clearance was equal to the glomerular filtration rate, but it is now known that it is less than that of inulin as urea is reabsorbed by the kidney tubules. In other medulla most of the increase in osmolality of the interstitial fluid is contributed by sodium chloride. It is in the inner medulla that sodium chloride and urea make an equal contribution.

## Answers and Explanations Practice Exam 4

**32 A C**
The number of glomeruli in the two kidneys is 2.5 x $10^6$. Each glomerulus is formed by a tuft of capillaries in the blunt end of the nephron. The afferent arteriole is slightly larger than the efferent. The capillary pressure in the glomeruli is probably some 40 mm Hg higher than in the pulmonary circulation which is a low pressure circulation.

**33 A B C**
The majority of filtered sodium is reabsorbed in the proximal tubule by active transport, the movement of sodium being accompanied by chloride. The rate of reabsorption is influenced by the filtered load so that glomerulo-tubular balance exists. The main hormone controlling sodium is aldosterone which acts on the distal convoluted tubule and collecting duct. The main action of vasopressin is on water reabsorption. It is chloride not sodium which is actively pumped out of the loop of Henle. Sodium reabsorption is also affected by physical factors influencing transport across capillary beds, notably hydrostatic pressure and plasma colloid osmotic pressure.

**34 A B D**
The contrast media for X-ray urography usually contain iodine. The material is freely filtered at the glomerulus but not secreted in the distal tubule.

**35 A C D**
Progesterone exerts its effect at the cell nucleus and the overall effect is catabolic. In general terms the action of progesterone is similar to that of oestrogen, but its thrust is to cause further differentiation of cells already primed with oestrogen. Thus the proliferative endometrium is converted to the glycogen-laden secretory endometrium suitable for implantation of a blastocyst. Oestrogen, not progesterone is produced as a result of androgen breakdown. Progesterone concentrations are elevated in pregnancy and fall towards term. The hormone can cross the placenta.

**36 A B**
In clinical hyperthyroidism (Graves' disease) the increased thyroid hormone release may result from a thyroidal antibody which exerts effects similar to those of TSH. However the TSH concentrations themselves are low in these patients. The elevated concentration of thyroid hormone in the plasma leads to an increased heart rate and oxygen consumption.

*Answers and Explanations Practice Exam 4*

**37 A B C D E**
Elevated growth hormone secretion results in gigantism in children in whom the epiphyses of the long bones have not fused and acromegaly in the adult. Release is also influenced by the composition of plasma, especially plasma glucose, release being stimulated when blood glucose concentrations fall. Release is increased during stress and exercise.

**38 C E**
Initiation of a nerve impulse is an all or none phenomenon. The magnitude is not dependent on the size of the stimulus. When the impulse reaches a particular region the membrane becomes permeable to sodium ions which enter the nerve fibre and the membrane depolarises, the potential inside changing from $-70mV$ to $+40mV$. Nerve impulses can travel equally well in either direction, but in the living animal conduction is normally in one direction as the fibre is only stimulated from one end. The conduction velocity increases with increased fibre diameter and is slowed by demyelination.

**39 A C E**
An EPSP represents depolarisation of the postsynaptic membrane produced by acetylcholine liberated from the pre-synaptic endings. It appears that acetylcholine causes short circuiting of the postsynaptic membrane by simultaneous increases in permeability to both sodium and potassium ions. Summation is seen and is important in integration in the central nervous system. EPSPs are involved in the stretch reflex.

**40 A D**
Following denervation of a mixed nerve there is flaccid paralysis of the muscle supplied as in the lower motor lesion. The sweat glands are also denervated. As the sympathetic fibres are cut, removing the tonic vasoconstriction, there will be vasodilatation and the area will be warmer. Of course sensation is lost. The central ends of cut fibres will regenerate.

**41 A B C E**
Cigarette smoking causes an increased risk of bladder cancer. $\beta$ naphthylamine was used in the rubber industry until it became apparent that it causes bladder cancer. Schistosomiasis and diverticula both predispose to bladder cancer, probably because both cause long-standing urinary infection, and the bacteria cause cancer via the nitrosamines they produce.

## Answers and Explanations Practice Exam 4

**42 A B C D E**
Tubular carcinomas are well differentiated tumours consisting of well-formed tubular structures. Lobular carcinomas are derived from cells of breast lobules; duct carcinomas from ducts; medullary carcinomas are characterised by a marked lymphoid infiltrate and a well-defined margin. Adenoid cystic carcinomas are rare primary carcinomas of the breast.

**43 B D E**
Cushing's syndrome is associated with osteoporosis. There may be left ventricular hypertrophy due to Cushing's-induced hypertension, and Kimmelstiel-Wilson renal lesions due to Cushing's-induced diabetes mellitus.

**44 B D E**
Renal stones are a feature of cystinuria and xanthinuria, inborn errors of metabolism. Hyperuricaemia, whether primary or secondary, predisposes to renal stone formation.

**45 A B C E**
Bone infarction is 'avascular necrosis'. It is associated with high dose steroids, irradiation, barotrauma, sickle cell disease, etc. In osteochondritis juvenilis the affected bone is infarcted, and this is believed to result from trauma to the bone which interferes with epiphyseal blood supply.

**46 C D**
Thiamine cannot be synthesised by animals, but is plentiful in wheat germ, oatmeal and yeast. Deficiency causes encephalopathy (Wernicke's), motor and sensory polyneuropathy and cardiomyopathy. Pellagra is caused by nicotinamide deficiency.

**47 A B C D E**
Polycystic disease present at birth is inherited as an autosomal recessive condition. Adult polycystic disease presents as renal failure, haematuria, heart failure, hypertension, or as an abdominal mass.

**48 B C**
The Guthrie test for phenylketonuria uses a mutant strain of $\beta$ *subtilis* which requires phenylalanine for growth.

## Answers and Explanations Practice Exam 4

**49 A B D E**
The defect in sickle cell disease lies in the replacement of HbA by HbS. HbS has a valine in place of glutamic acid in the sixth amino acid residue of the $\beta$ chains of the globin molecule. In sickle anaemia there is a haemolytic anaemia, which is associated with bone marrow hyperplasia and increased serum iron levels. Bone infarcts are common.

**50 A C D**
Nephroblastomas commonly contain mesenchymal elements such as striated muscle, in addition to primitive glomeruli and renal tubules; neuroblastomas consist of neuroblasta; teratomas contain ectoderm, mesoderm and endoderm.

**51 A B C E**
In Hodgkin's disease the normal lymph node architecture is replaced by a mixed population of cells including eosinophils, plasma cells, fibroblasts, lymphocytes and characteristically, Reed-Sternberg cells. Asteroid bodies are inclusions in macrophage giant cells.

**52 A**
The Schick test consists of an injection of diphtheria toxin into the skin - a negative reaction demonstrates the presence of neutralising antitoxin. The Dick test is appropriate for streptococcal immunity; the Frei test for lymphogranuloma; the Kveim for sarcoidosis. Coombs described a fluorescent antibody technique.

**53 A B C E**
Secondary hyperparathyroidism is a common sequel to chronic renal failure. Renal stones are the most common mode of presentation of hyperparathyroidism. Osteomalacia is caused by vitamin D deficiency. Carcinoma of the parathyroid gland is a very rare cause of hyperparathyroidism.

**54 B C D E**
The gene for haemophilia, recessive and carried on the X chromosome, will be passed by the father to all his daughters, none of whom will therefore be normal. An average of half the sons and half the daughters of such marriages will have clinical haemophilia.

**55 A B D**
Transplacental transfer of antibody, and diphtheria antitoxin administration represent examples of passive immunisation.

## Answers and Explanations Practice Exam 4

**56 A C**
Sternal pain and tenderness are common in acute leukaemias. Chloromas are tumours consisting of myeloblasts. A high proportion of cases of acute lymphoblastic leukaemias are cured by chemotherapy. Haemorrhagic tendency is best corrected by platelet transfusion.

**57 C D**
Inflammation starts in the synovial membrane, with accumulations of inflammatory cells. This inflammatory tissue (pannus) gradually encroaches on the cartilage margins, erodes the cartilage and replaces it with fibrous tissue. Granulomas are not seen in rheumatoid arthritis. Fibrillation of cartilage is seen in osteoarthritis.

**58 A B C D**
Aplastic anaemia may develop secondary to many drugs either predictably (with folic acid antagonist and other cytotoxic agents) or idiosynchratically (eg. phenylbutazone). It can rarely be seen in miliary tuberculosis and is frequently part of the natural history of paroxysmal nocturnal haemoglobinuria, when the aplasia may be transient or long-lasting. Zeive's syndrome is an acute transient hyperlipaemia (due to hepatopancreatic damage) after a drinking bout. The condition improves on withdrawal of alcohol.

**59 B D**
Myeloid or giant cell epulis is a reactive swelling of gums. Glomus tumours are tumours of temperature-sensitive arteriovenous anastamoses, mostly situated in the skin. Ameloblastomas arise in the jaw bone from tooth precursors. Wilm's tumour arises in the kidney (nephroblastoma); Ewing's sarcoma is a tumour arising in bone in children, and consists of small round undifferentiated cells.

**60 D E**
Perforation is rare in Crohn's disease: transmural inflammation causes adhesions, and fissuring ulceration then produces fistulae. Neuronal hyperplasia in the muscularis propria is common.

125

# ANSWERS TO EXAM 5

**1 D E**

The inguinal canal is 3-4 cm long. The conjoint tendon is in the medial part of the posterior wall. The ilio-inguinal nerve, as it passes just superior to the inguinal ligament deep to the external oblique, enters the inguinal canal and emerges through the superficial ring. The genital branch of the genitofemoral nerve enters the canal through the deep ring and supplies the cremaster muscle. The inguinal ligament forms the floor of the canal with its lacunar ligament at its medial end between the ligament and the pubic bone.

**2 A B C D E**

The pelvic fascial covering is separated from the prostatic capsule by a venous plexus. Lymphatic vessels from the prostate go to the external and internal iliac and sacral nodes. The pelvic veins communicate with the vertebral venous plexuses and thus with all levels of the trunk and the intracranial venous sinuses.

**3 B C**

The splanchnic nerves are medial to the ganglionated trunk. The least (lowest) splanchnic nerves go to the renal ganglia. Postganglionic sympathetic fibres come from the lumbar (and sacral) ganglia and go to the viscera as well as the postganglionic fibres from the preaortic ganglia in which most of the splanchnic nerves end.

**4 A B**

The pudendal nerve leaves the pelvis by passing through the greater sciatic foramen inferior to the piriformis muscle. It crosses the ischial spine where it is medial to the internal pudendal vessels and enters the perineum through the lesser sciatic foramen. It runs forwards in the pudendal (Alcock's) canal on the lateral wall of the ischiorectal fossa and is the main sensory nerve to the skin and muscles of the perineum. The internal anal sphincter consists of smooth muscle and has an autonomic nerve suply. The skin over the symphysis pubis is supplied by the 1st lumbar spinal nerve, mainly through the ilio-inguinal.

**5 C E**

The ductus arteriosus passes between the left pulmonary artery and the arch of the aorta. It develops from the 6th aortic arch. The recurrent laryngeal nerve hooks round the 6th arch which mostly disappears on the right so that the right nerve hooks round the 4th arch (the subclavian artery) because the 5th aortic arch disappears on both sides. On the left, the 6th arch persists as the pulmonary trunk and ductus arteriosus. It is thought that the blood from the

## Answers and Explanations Practice Exam 5

superior vena cava eventually passes through the ductus arteriosus and that from the inferior vena cava through the foramen ovale of the intra-atrial septum. Increased intra-aortic pressure and decreased pressure in the pulmonary artery reverses the flow of the blood but the actual closure is due largely to contraction of muscle in the wall of the ductus. Coarctation of the aorta occurs just proximal or distal to the ductus or opposite the ductus and is classified accordingly.

**6 A C D E**
The pancreas develops from the foregut as a smaller ventral and a larger dorsal diverticulum. The ventral part rotates and joins the dorsal part. The superior mesenteric artery at its commencement is posterior to the neck of the pancreas. As it passes downwards it lies in front of the uncinate process.

**7 A C**
The opening to the inferior vena cava is at the level of the 8th thoracic vertebra and also transmits the right phrenic nerve. The attachment of the central tendon to the fibrous pericardium accounts for changes in the position and shape of the heart during respiration. The sympathetic trunk is posterior to the medial arcuate ligament and the subcostal nerve is posterior to the lateral.

**8 A D**
The dorsalis pedis artery, a continuation of the anterior tibial, leaves the dorsum of the foot through the proximal end of the 1st intermetatarsal space. It is most easily palpable at this point. The tendon of the tibialis anterior muscle is attached to the medial cuneiform and the base of the first metatarsal. The peroneal trochlea separates the tendons of the peroneus longus and brevis muscles and the peroneus longus is inferior to the trochlea.

**9 D E**
The capsule of the hip joint is attached anteriorly to the intertrochanteric line and posteriorly to the neck 1 cm medial to the crest. The main source of blood to the head of the femur in the adult is from the blood vessels entering its neck from the retinacula of the capsule. In the child the ligament of the head is important. The iliofemoral ligament is attached to the anterior inferior iliac spine.

**10 A B**
The ulnar nerve passes backwards at the level of the middle of the upper arm and continues downwards in front of the medial head of the triceps brachii muscle to the elbow where the nerve lies in a

## Answers and Explanations Practice Exam 5

groove on the back of the medial epicondyle. The nerve enters the forearm by passing forwards between the heads of the flexor carpi ulnaris. It enters the hand superficial to the flexor retinaculum and is lateral to the pisiform bone and medial to the hook of the hamate. Its dorsal branch is given off about 5 cm above the level of the wrist.

**11 B C D**
The pharyngeal branch of the vagus nerve is motor to the muscles of the pharynx, except the stylopharyngeus, and the muscles of the palate except the tensor veli palatini. Its superior laryngeal branch divides into the external laryngeal nerve, which supplies the cricothyroid muscle, and the internal laryngeal nerve which is sensory to the larynx above the vocal folds. The right recurrent laryngeal nerve is given off in the neck, supplies the rest of the laryngeal muscles and is sensory to the larynx below the vocal folds.

**12 C D**
The posterior triangle is bounded by the trapezius (posterior) and sternocleidomastoid (anterior) muscles. Superiorly they almost meet at the superior nuchal line. The inferior belly of the omohyoid muscle crosses its floor. The trunks of the brachial plexus are inferior to the omohyoid and the upper trunk gives off the suprascapular nerve. There are two layers of fascia roofing over the triangle - a superficial from the investing layer and a deep from the prevertebral part of the cervical fascia. The accessory nerve runs between the two layers.

**13 A C**
The thymus develops from the endoderm of the 3rd pharyngeal pouch at the cranial end of the foregut. It is distinctly lobulated due to its fibrous septa. It does not decrease in size until puberty. The thymic corpuscles consist of degenerating epithelial elements and their function is not known.

**14 A D**
The horizontal part of the duodenum is anterior to the right psoas muscle, right ureter, inferior vena cava, gonadal vessels and abdominal aorta. It is crossed anteriorly by the mesentery and superior mesenteric vessels. It is at the level of the 3rd lumbar vertebra.

**15 B C**
The thoraco-acromial artery arises medial to the pectoralis minor and its branches pierce the clavipectoral fascia. The cephalic vein also pierces this fascia and joins the axillary vein. The basilic vein joins the brachial veins to form the axillary vein. The radial nerve passes behind the humerus in its groove (spiral groove).

## Answers and Explanations Practice Exam 5

**16 A B C**
There is a space between the scalanus anterior (lateral) and longus colli (medial) in which are found the vertebral and inferior thyroid arteries, the sympathetic trunk, inferior cervical ganglion and ventral rami of the 7th and 8th cervical spinal nerves. The arteries are anterior to the nerves and the inferior thyroid artery is anterior to the vertebral.

**17 B**
The spinous process of the atlas is represented by a tubercle. The anterior arch is much smaller than the posterior. The rectus capitis posterior major muscle is attached to the spine of the axis and the occipital bone. An alar ligament is attached to the dens of the axis and the medial side of the occipital condyle.

**18 A B E**
The mental branch of the inferior alveolar (dental) nerve, a branch of the mandibular, supplies the auriculotemporal nerve the lower lip and side of the scalp. The infraorbital nerve, a branch of the maxillary, supplies the skin of the lower eyelid. There are usually no sensory branches of the 1st cervical nerve. This applies to both its ventral and dorsal rami. The greater occipital and 3rd occipital nerves are branches of the dorsal rami of the 2nd and 3rd cervical nerves respectively and supply the back of the scalp.

**19 A C D**
The gubernaculum testis is homologous with the ovarian and round ligaments (gubernaculum ovarii). The ductus deferens corresponds with the duct of epoophoron (of Gartner) both being derived from the mesonephric (Wolffian) duct. The paramesonephric (Mullerian) duct forms the uterine tube, uterus and part of the vagina. In the male it is represented by the appendix of the testis and the prostatic utricle. The female urthral glands correspond with the prostatic glands.

**20 A D E**
There is a plexus of postganglionic sympathetic fibres round the artery derived mainly from the stellate ganglion. The vertebral artery is anterior to the spinal accessory nerve as they enter the skull through the foramen magnum. The vertebral artery supplies the spinal cord with cervical segmental branches and long descending branches. The vertebral artery gives off the important posterior inferior cerebellar artery; the basilar artery gives off another two cerebellar arteries.

## Answers and Explanations Practice Exam 5

**21 A B D E**
Reflex vasoconstriction follows blood loss, baroreceptors in the aortic arch and carotid sinuses being involved. Baroreceptors may also be influenced by carotid occlusion which reduces pressure in the region of the receptors. Massive sympathetic outflow associated with asphyxia also results in vasoconstriction. Baroreceptors are involved in a Valsalva manoeuvre when the return of blood to the heart is greatly reduced so that the arterial blood presure falls. Venous return improves on lying down so that no compensatory vasoconstriction is seen.

**22 A B C E**
Sympathetic stimulation causes an increase in heart rate through an action on the sino-atrial node. There is also a shift in the Starling curve to the left with increased myocardial contractility. The increased myocardial contractility leads to an increased oxygen consumption and an increased cardiac output. There is also increased coronary blood flow.

**23 C D E**
Carbon dioxide dissolves in plasma to form carbonic acid which dissociates to form bicarbonate, the main form in which carbon dioxide is transported, but not in the erythrocyte. It also forms a neutral carbamino compound with haemoglobin and combines to a lesser extent with plasma proteins. The partial pressure $CO_2$ is 40 mmHg (5kPa) in arterial blood and 46 mmHG (6kPa) in venous blood.

**24 A B C D**
Following the period of isometric contraction of the ventricles the aortic and pulmonary valves open, blood is ejected and the pressure in the ventricles drops. The pressure in the aorta is now greater than in the left ventricle and the aortic, as well as the pulmonary valves, close, giving the second heart sound. Ventricular filling occurs in diastole and the atrial pressure is slightly higher than the ventricular pressure, otherwise the blood would not enter the ventricles. Thus the thin walled atria do not merely act as venous reservoirs, but their contraction produces small but important changes in atrial pressure.

**25 B D E**
The medullary respiratory centre is thought to comprise inspiratory and expiratory neurones which to an extent intermingle. The respiratory centre is thought to have inherent rhythmicity which is not dependent on higher centres. The activity is influenced by neural

## Answers and Explanations Practice Exam 5

inputs from many regions including the limbic system and hypothalamus. Pain can provide a potent stimulus of respiration, leading to marked hypocapnia and alkalosis. Respiration is also stimulated centrally by an increase in the $pCO_2$ or increase in the hydrogen ion concentration of the blood.

**26 A C**
Abnormal matching of ventilation and blood flow as in emphysema results in a fall in arterial $pO_2$. A decrease in the oxygen tension of the blood also results from ascent to altitude. Decreased alveolar ventilation resulting from a multitude of factors including increased airway resistance leads to a fall in arterial $pO_2$. Carriage of oxygen is influenced by the haemoglobin concentration and by the combination of haemoglobin with carbon monoxide, but the arterial $pO_2$ is unaffected in these situations.

**27 E**
Hyperkalaemia occurs in patients with renal failure. Potassium concentrations may be returned to normal quite rapidly by infusing glucose with insulin. Insulin causes potassium to enter the cells and the plasma potassium is reduced. Additional infusion of glucose is given to prevent its plasma concentration from falling also. Chlorpropamide is used in the treatment of diabetes.

**28 C**
Intrinsic factor is secreted by the parietal cells of the stomach and aids in the absorption of cyanocobalamin (vitimin $B_{12}$) in the terminal ileum. It is not involved in the absorption of folic acid even though it is part of the $B_{12}$ complex. Injections of $B_{12}$ have no effect on the production of intrinsic factor.

**29 C D E**
Active transport is an energy dependent process linked to aerobic and anaerobic metabolism. When cells stop actively adjusting the distribution of ions across the cell membrane excess water enters the cells which swell. Glucose is absorbed rapidly in the small intestine by two independent mechanisms, diffusion and active transport. Active transport is also involved with hydrogen ion secretion by the kidney.

**30 A B**
In some people especially children, the ganglia of the intrinsic plexuses of part of the distal colon or rectum degenerate. The defaecation reflex fails and the colon above the affected part becomes enormously distended. The majority of water reabsorption in the gastro-intestinal tract does not occur in the colon.

## Answers and Explanations Practice Exam 5

**31 B C E**
Blood glucose in prolonged fasting is maintained at a level of 2.5 mmol/1, or half that normally seen, by various mechanisms including liver gluconeogenesis which is promoted by the fall in insulin concentrations.

**32 A B D E**
Fluid passes out of the capillaries at the arterial end under the influence of hydrostatic pressure and returns to the venous circulation as a result of the oncotic pressure exerted by the plasma proteins. If there is an increase in filtration pressure occurring, as for example with increased capillary pressure, additional fluid passes into the tissue. If there is a reduction in plasma osmotic pressure as in liver disease when there is a fall in albumin synthesis, then there is a reduction in the amount of fluid returning to the circulation. Under normal circumstances excess tissue fluid may be removed by the lymphatics. Obstruction of these vessels results in oedema.

**33 D E**
Obligatory absorption of salt and water - 7/8ths of the filtered load occurs in the proximal tubule. The major force for filtrate absorption is active reabsorption of sodium; chloride follows passively. It is in the loop of Henle that active chloride absorption is the driving force. The main site of action of aldosterone is in the distal tubule. Both PAH and hydrogen ions are actively secreted in the proximal tubule.

**34 A**
The cause of respiratory acidosis is increased arterial $pCO_2$ with an accompanying increase in $H^+$. It arises from conditions which impair the efficiency of gas exchange in the lungs such as pneumonia or respiratory depression. A fully compensated acidosis is one in which the pH of the blood has been restored to normal via the kidney which adds bicarbonate to the blood. Hence the plasma bicarbonate is raised.

**35 B E**
The main hormones secreted by the anterior pituitary are growth hormone (somatotrophin), prolactin, the gonadotrophins, LH and FSH, thyrotrophin and ACTH. Somatostatin (growth hormone release inhibiting hormone) is synthesised in the hypothalamus and many other regions. Oxytocin is a posterior pituitary hormone and aldosterone is produced in the adrenal cortex.

## Answers and Explanations Practice Exam 5

**36  A B C**
In the first half of the cycle the developing follicles, under the influence of FSH, secrete oestradiol, which causes proliferation of the endometrium and its blood vessels. Mid-cycle, the mucous becomes thinner, facilitating transport of sperm, and there is an increase in body temperature. Although the second half of the cycle is called the secretory phase, gonadotrophins are not secreted by the endometrium. They are of pituitary origin (or in the case of pregnancy also of placental origin).

**37  B C E**
The normal plasma calcium is generally 2.5 mM of which about 50% exists in the ionised form. Low calcium diminishes release of calcitonin and causes hyperexcitation of nerves, which is the cause of tetany, also seen with hyperventilation. Low vitamin D interferes with calcium absorption. A primary defect in parathyroid hormone output results in a fall in plasma calcium.

**38  B C E**
Glucagon is a polypeptide hormone secreted by the $a_2$ cells of the pancreatic islands. It influences carbohydrate metabolism, catalysing liver phosphorylation, the first step in glycogenolysis. Consistent with its effects on carbohydrate metabolism is the fact that release is stimulated by a fall in blood glucose concentrations as in fasting. Glucagon stimulates insulin production.

**39  A C D**
The sympathetic nerves supply sweat glands, arterioles, dilator pupillae and eyelids. The sympathetic nervous supply maintains vasoconstrictor tone, so that damage to the supply leads to vasodilatation. Stimulation of the sympathetic system leads to midriasis (dilation of the pupil) and paralysis to miosis (constriction of the pupil). There is no innervation by the sympathetic of the ciliary muscle so paralysis leads to no effect on the ability to accommodate.

133

## Answers and Explanations Practice Exam 5

**40 A B C E**
The convection currents induced in the semicircular canals as a result of introducing cold water into the external meatus of the ear cause nystagmus, twisting of the trunk and a feeling of giddiness. Thus it is unwise to syringe out the external auditory meatus with water not at 37°C. It takes some 20 sec. or more for eye movements to be produced. It is the slow phase of nystagmus which is towards the affected side as cold endolymph is dense and so tends to fall, which is the same movement as producing rotation of the nose away from the affected side. To stabilise the visual image, lateral deviation of the gaze towards the cooled side is indicated. Eye reflexes are seen in unconscious patients providing the brain stem is functioning. The test can be used in diagnosis of lesion of the vestibular apparatus and its connections.

**41 None correct**
Conn's syndrome is caused by aldosterone-secreting adenomas of the adrenal cortex. Cushing's syndrome is usually due to hyperplasia or adenomas of the adrenal cortex, while carcinoma accounts for approximately 10%. Acromegaly is due to acidophil adenomas of the pituitary. Paroxysmal hypertension is associated with phaeochromocytoma, usually benign. Hyperparathyroidism is only rarely due to a carcinoma.

**42 A E**
Cerebral infarction may occur due to embolus from a mural thrombus or due to hypotension.

**43 A E**
Molluscum sebaceum, also known as Keratoacanthoma, is a benign tumour of unknown aetiology which macroscopically and microscopically may be mistaken for a squamous carcinoma. These lesions heal spontaneously within a few months.

**44 A B**
Metastatic calcification is seen in association with increased levels of calcium (or occasionally with increased phosphate) in blood and tissues, when normal tissues become calcified.

*Answers and Explanations Practice Exam 5*

**45  A D**
When a nucleus contains two X chromosomes, only one is expressed; the other becomes condensed and, in neutrophils, appears as a protrusion from the nucleus: a 'Barr body'. Normal females, and patients with Klinefelter's disease (XXY) thus have Barr bodies, while males, and patients with Turner's syndrome (XO) have none. In chronic granulocytic leukaemia there is deletion of the long arm of chromosome 22 (Ph$^1$ chromosome).

**46  A C**
Mitral stenosis, pulmonary hypertension and atrial septal defects predispose to right ventricular failure.

**47  C E**
The osmotic diuresis of diabetic ketosis causes water depletion and loss of potassium ions. The plasma potassium level is commonly raised, however, (probably due to poor glucose entry into cells), but falls rapidly with therapy. There is a metabolic acidosis with compensatory respiratory alkalosis.

**48  A B D**
A colour-blind girl has an abnormal gene on each X chromosome, and her father must have supplied one (he is also colour-blind). Since cystic fibrosis is autosomal recessive, the mother carries an abnormal gene. The gene causing haemophilia in a boy is on the X chromosome, always from the mother. Familial polyposis is an autosomal dominant condition, and the gene may derive from either parent.

**49  C D E**
Pernicious anaemia is a syndrome caused by diminished gastric secretion of intrinsic factor, and therefore vitamin $B_{12}$ absorption. Deficiency of vitamin $B_{12}$ may occasionally be caused by the malabsorption syndrome or by the fish tapeworm, which competes for available $B_{12}$. $B_{12}$ deficiency causes reduced production of all cells, including red and white blood cells and platelets, and mucosal cells (glossitis and diarrhoea).

**50  B**
Meningiomas occur most often between 40 and 60 years of age. Medulloblastomas occur only in children. Appendical carcinoids occur at any age. Chondrosarcomas are commoner in later life; teratomas are seen predominantly in young adults.

## Answers and Explanations Practice Exam 5

**51 B E**
Reticulocytes are red cells which are still producing haemoglobin, relatively immature, and their presence in increased numbers generally denotes increased or ineffective bone marrow production and release of erythrocytes.

**52 B D**
In most cases chromosome 22 has part of its long arm deleted and translocated to chromosome 9. It has a peak incidence at 40-50 years, and is rare below 20. The marrow is hyperplastic, with increased numbers of both mature and immature cells. The white cells typically show a very low alkaline phosphatase.

**53 A D E**
Amyloidosis may complicate any disease in which there is longstanding inflammation (Hodgkin's disease shows many of the features of a chronic inflammatory disease). Amyloid is produced by the tumour cells of medullary carcinoma of thyroid.

**54 B D**
The convention is that the normal range encompasses 95% of the population under study, thus excluding 2.5% at each extreme. This represents the mean±2 standard deviations.

**55 A B D E**
Rickettsiae resemble bacteria in possessing both RNA and DNA, but are, like viruses, obligate intracellular parasites unable to reproduce without the aid of host cells. They are generally gram negative, but are better stained by Giemsa. They are sensitive to many antibiotics, but only the tetracyclines and chloramphenicol are sufficiently potent to be of therapeutic value.

**56 A D E**
*S.aureus* may produce an enterotoxin when it grows in food. Many strains of *Cl. welchii*, an organism normally present in the intestine, contaminate meat in the slaughterhouse and will multiply and produce toxins if the meat becomes warm and anaerobic. *Cl. botulinum* is a soil saphrophyte which produces an extremely potent and frequently lethal exotoxin when it grows in food.

*Answers and Explanations Practice Exam 5*

**57  A B D E**
Ova hatch in warm wet soil and develop into embryos which enter the skin, reach the lungs through the venous system and migrate up bronchi to the oesophagus. They reach the intestine and mature as worms attached to the mucosa, which shed ova into the faeces. Ankylostoma infestation is common in tropical and subtropical countries, and is second only to malaria as a world producer of death and chronic ill-health.

**58  C**
Injection of live attenuated organisms (Bacillus-Calmette-Guerin) is the best method of conferring resistance to tuberculosis.

**59  A E**
Osteoarthritis is characterised by fibrillation of cartilage, followed by complete cartilage loss, and osteophyte formation at the joint periphery. Lymphoid follicles are seen in rheumatoid arthritis.

**60  B C D**
Acanthosis nigricans is associated with internal malignancy (eg. stomach, pancreas, lung). Leukoplakia means a white patch on a mucous membrane, which microscopically may be due to hyperplasia, hyperkeratosis and varying degrees of atypia. Solar keratosis is a hyperkeratotic lesion induced by prolonged skin exposure, and a proportion of these progress to squamous carcinoma. Bowen's disease is an in-situ squamous carcinoma of the skin.

# READING & REFERENCE BOOKS

Anderson, J. R. **Muirs Textbook of Pathology** 5th edition 1979 pub. Churchill Livingstone.

Basmajian, J. V. **Grants Method of Anatomy** 10th edition pub. Williams and Williams.

Bell, G. H. Emslie-Smith, D. & Paterson, C. R. **Textbook of Physiology** pub. Churchill Livingstone 1980.

Ganong, W. F. **Review of Medical Physiology** 11th edition pub. Lange Medical Publications 1983.

Gillies, R. R. **Lecture Notes in Medical Microbiology** 2nd edition pub. Blackwell 1978.

Goodman, L. S. & Gilman, A. **The Pharmacological Basis of therapeutics** 7th edition pub. MacMillan 1985.

Gray, C. H. & Howarth, P. J. N. **Clinical Chemical Pathology** 9th edition pub. Edward Arnold 1979.

Hughes Jones, N. C. **Lecture Notes in Haematology** 4th edition pub. Blackwell 1984.

Kelman, G. R. **Physiology: A Clinical Approach** 3rd edition pub. Churchill Livingstone 1980.

McMinn, R. M. H. & Hutchings, R. T. **Colour Atlas of Anatomy** pub. Wolfe, Medical Publishers 1978.

Moore, K. L. **Clinically Oriented Anatomy** pub. Williams Wilkins 1980.

Mountcastle, V. B. **Medical Physiology** 14th edition pub. Mosby 1980.

Walter, O. B. & Israel, M. S. **General Pathology** 5th edition pub. Churchill Livingstone 1979.

# MCQ REVISION INDEX

This index contains a list of the principal topics, conditions, structures and diseases mentioned in these practice exams. Each item in the Index is followed by a number which refers to a specific question in one of the practice exams, ie 3.27 indicates Practice Exam 3 question number 27.

## A
actin 3.39
actinomyces israelii 1.59
active immunisation 4.55
active transport 5.29
adenocarcinoma
  prostate 3.54
adenolymphoma 3.46
adipose tissue cells 2.28
adrenal corticosteroids 2.35
airways resistance 2.25
aldosterone 1.35
alpha-fetoprotein 1.47
amyloid 2.55
amyloidosis 5.53
ankylostoma 5.57
aorta
  syphilitic disease 1.53
aortic arch 2.19
aortic valve 3.21
arm 5.15
artery
  aortic arch 4.20
  inferior epigastric 4.08
  left coronary 1.02
  radial 2.01
  right coronary 3.17
  ulnar 1.09
  vertebral 5.20
arthritis
  osteoarthritis 5.59
  rheumatoid 4.57
ascites 2.60
aspartate transaminase 2.59
atheroma 1.58
atlas 5.17
axilla 2.03

## B
bacteroides 1.45
Barr bodies 5.45
Berry aneurysms 2.51

blood
  volume 3.27
blood pressure
  systemic 4.21
bone marrow failure 4.58
brachial plexus 1.03
breast 4.10
burns
  shock treatment 1.21

## C
calcification
  metastatic 5.44
capillaries 3.23
carbon dioxide 2.24; 5.23
carcinoma
  bladder 4.41
  breast 4.42
  colonic 1.57
  larynx 2.52
  risks 3.53
cardiac cycle 5.24
cardiac output 2.21
cerebellum 1.39; 4.02
chemical transmitter 2.38
Cheyne-Stokes respiration 4.26
chordae tendinae 3.21
cirrhosis 1.52
clotting 4.23
coeliac disease 3.29
creatine kinase 3.56
Crohn's disease 3.52; 4.60
Cushing's syndrome 4.43
cutaneous malignancy 5.60
cytoplasmic receptors 3.36

## D
deep perineal space 2.11
dehydration
  secondary 1.33
diabetes mellitus 1.36
diabetic ketosis 5.47

diaphragm 2.07; 5.07
  pelvic 2.15
diphtheria 4.52
diverticulosis 3.49
Down's syndrome 2.53
drugs 2.43
ductus arteriosus 5.05
duodenum 5.14

# E
ear 3.12
ECG 3.24
elbow 2.09
embryo 1.19; 3.06
endometrium 5.36
excitatory postsynaptic potential 4.39
exercise 3.28
external auditory meatus 5.40
extracellular fluid volume 3.33
eyeball 3.11; 4.06

# F
fasting 5.31
femoral triangle 1.17; 4.17
Fick principle 2.21
fingers 3.16
food poisoning 5.56
foot 5.08
foramen magnum 4.14
fossa
  ischiorectal 2.12
  popliteal 2.10
functional residual capacity 3.26

# G
gall bladder 1.08
gastrectomy 2.31
gastric secretion 2.29
genes 5.48
gland
  parotid 2.14
  pituitary 3.08
  prostate 3.15; 5.02
glucagon 5.38
glucose 3.32
gluten-sensitive enteropathy 3.29
Graves' disease 4.36
growth hormone 4.37
Guthrie test 4.48

# H
haemoglobin
  oxygen 3.22
haemolytic anaemia 1.41
haemophilia 4.54
haemorrhage
  intracerebral 1.55
hand
  bones 1.10
heart 3.09
  sympathetic nerves 5.22
herpes zoster 3.45
hip joint 5.09
Hodgkin's disease 4.51
hydrocephalus 2.57
hydrogen ions 1.28
hypercholesterolaemia 3.43
hyperparathyroidism 4.53
hypertrophy
  left ventricular 1.56
hyperventilation 4.25
hypothalamus 2.04; 2.37

# I
IgM 3.41
ileum 4.29
immunisation 5.58
infarction 2.54
infectious mononucleosis 1.54
inguinal canal 1.16; 5.01
innervation
  face and scalp 5.18
inspiration 2.26
insulin 3.35
intrinsic factor 5.28

# K
kidney 3.32
  countercurrent multiplier system 1.32
  drug excretion 2.33
  glomeruli 4.32
  sodium 4.33
  urea 4.31
knee jerk 2.39

# MCQ Revision Index

## L
left ventricular failure  5.46
leukaemia  2.41
  acute lymphoblastic  4.56
  chronic lymphatic  3.48; 3.60
  chronic myeloid  5.52
liver  4.27
lung compliance  1.26

## M
mandible  1.01
medullary carcinoma of thyroid  2.46
megacolon  5.30
meninges  1.18
menstrual cycle  5.36
metabolic rate  1.27
midgut
  in embryo  3.18
  structures  2.02
molluscum sebaceum  5.43
mucosal lining  1.29
muscle
  biceps femoris  3.05
  deltoid  3.07
  obturator internus  4.05
  psoas major  2.20
  rectus abdominis  4.03
  scalenus anterior  5.16
  skeletal  3.39
myocardial infarction  5.42

## N
necrosis
  avascular  4.45
neoplasms  5.50
  of bone  1.43
nephrotic syndrome  3.55
nerve
  action potential  4.38
  common peroneal  2.13
  femoral  4.19
  glossopharyngeal  3.02
  hypoglossal  1.11
  ilio-inguinal  2.17
  left phrenic  4.07
  median  1.14; 4.12
  obturator  4.13
  pelvic splanchnic  2.18
  pudendal  5.04
  radial  3.10
  right vagus  5.11
  sciatic  3.04; 4.15
  section  4.40
  splanchnic  5.03
  ulnar  5.10
nerve fibres
  preganglionic sympathetic  3.20
nervous system
  autonomic  1.15
  sympathetic  1.07
normal range  5.54

## O
oedema  4.22; 5.32
oesophagus  1.06
oestradiol  5.36
oestrogen  3.37
omentum
  lesser  4.04
oral contraceptives  3.37
orbit  1.13; 2.06
osmotic diuretics  1.34
oxygen  1.25; 5.26
oxygen-haemoglobin  2.23

## P
pancreas  4.28; 5.06
parathyroid hormone  2.36
pericardium
  serous  2.08
perineal body  1.12
perineal pouch
  superficial  3.13
peripheral resistance  1.22
pernicious anaemia  5.49
phenylketonuria  3.57
pituitary
  anterior pituitary  5.35
  basophil adenoma  1.48
plasma
  calcium  5.37
  magnesium  1.44
  potassium  5.27
  proteins  2.27
polycythaemia  1.50; 2.45
polymorphonuclear leucocytes  1.60
posterior mediastinum  1.20
posterior triangle  5.12

primary gout 1.51
progesterone 3.37; 4.35
prolactin 1.38
proximal tubule 5.33
pseudomonas aeruginosa 1.46
pulmonary
  surfactant 3.25
  irritant receptors 1.24
pyloric stenosis 3.47

**R**
rectum 1.05
red cells
  hypochromic microcytic 3.42
renal stones 4.44
renal blood flow 2.32
renal disease
  polycystic 4.47
respiratory acidosis 5.34
respiratory centre 5.25
reticulocyte count 5.51
retina 2.40
retinoblastoma 2.48
rhesus factor 1.49; 2.22
rib 4.09
rickettsiae 5.55

**S**
scapula
  movements 4.16
Schaumann bodies 1.42
secretin 3.30
segmentation
  small intestine 3.31
sickle cell disease 4.49
silica 3.58
spermatic cord 3.03
spinal cord
  transection 3.40
spirochaetes 2.50
steatorrhoea 2.30
steroid hormones 3.36
stomach 2.16; 3.14
  arterial blood supply 1.04
  hunger contractions 1.30
streptococcus pyogenes 2.47; 3.44
supraoptic nucleus 3.38
swallowing 4.01
systemic filling pressure 1.23

**T**
T-lymphocytes 3.50
teeth eruption 3.19
teratomas 2.56
tetanus 3.59
thiamine 4.46
thrombocythaemia 2.49
thymus 5.13
thyroid binding globulin 1.37
treponemal infection 2.44
tropomyosin 3.39
tumours 3.51; 4.50
  bone 4.59
  malignant 5.41

**U**
ureter
  right 4.18
ureterocolic anastamosis 2.42
urine 3.34

**V**
vagina 4.11
vagotomy 4.30
vasoconstriction 5.21
vasodilatation 4.24
vasopressin 3.38
vein
  basilic 2.05

**W**
water 2.34
wrist
  bones 1.10
  flexor retinaculum 3.01

**X**
X-ray 4.34

**Z**
Zollinger-Ellison syndrome 1.31